Understanding Homœ
Homœopathic Unders

Julian Carlyon

Understanding Homœopathy,

Homœopathic Understanding

*Foundations of homœopathic
philosophy and practice*

Julian Carlyon

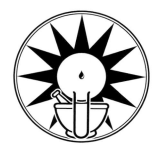

Helios Homoeopathy Ltd

Understanding Homœopathy, Homœopathic Understanding

First published in 2003 by Helios

© 2003 Julian Carlyon
Julian Carlyon has asserted his right under the Copyright, Designs and Patents Act 1988 to be identified as the Author of this Work.

Cover design, typesetting and illustrations by Dragon Design
Typeset in Lingwood 9.8/14.4 pt

ISBN 0-9530144-4-4

Printed in Italy

For our dear Adam

Table of Contents

Acknowledgements

My first thanks must go to the teachers, mentors and friends who have helped and inspired me along the way. Of these I'd like to especially acknowledge John Damonte, Misha Norland and Barbara Somers. Without their guidance this book would not have been possible.

Throughout the writing of the book I've received invaluable feedback and criticism from several dear friends and colleagues.

Special thanks go to Andrew Kirk, Peter Adams and Richard Vick for their sustained support and feedback. Valuable responses to my work also came from Guy Cooper, Martin Large, Veronica Meanwell, Sheila Ryan, Katherine Haggiag and Michael Haggiag.

Thanks also go to Fred Hageneder for thoughtful and creative design, and to Claudine Whiting for her careful editorial work. Special thanks must also go to John Morgan for his long-standing support for the project, and offer to publish.

Last but not least I thank my wife, Rissa, for her patience throughout the protracted birth of this book. Thanks also to the students, past and present, who shared the journey with me.

Introduction

Samuel Hahnemann conceived of homœopathy as a rational healing art. In other words homœopathy is based on readily understandable and clear principles available to all. However, this rationality must be watered and nourished with intuition. A *rational healing art* – this was Hahnemann's aim and desire.

He intended that the practitioner should be guided by simple yet profound truths. Truths that are at once profound and simple are also perennial. They appear ever and anew, dressed in the apparel of time and place.

Hahnemann formulated the conceptual framework of homœopathy at the end of the eighteenth and beginning of the nineteenth centuries. The seventeenth century saw the emergence of scientific empiricism out of the more imaginative Hermetic tradition of knowledge. Men of science such as Isaac Newton had a deep and abiding interest in the alchemical tradition – a tradition in which inner and outer, mind and matter were intuited to be but different aspects of a single reality.

Hahnemann, in embracing the new rationalism, was at the same time left without a map, without a conceptual framework, to describe his perception of the dynamic reality that lay behind the activity of both mind and body. Although a scientist, he reached back into the hermetic age to rescue the notion of vitalism in order to describe what he saw. His idea of the vital force was not new; simply a renewed expression of an idea that stretched back, via scientists such as Newton, via sixteenth century alchemists that preceded him, to Paracelsus and beyond. In doing this he put himself in a stream of ideas concerned with the possibility of transformation, not only of the human soul, but of substance as well.

At the end of the nineteenth century James Tyler Kent's homœopathic philosophy was imbued with the same thread of investigation and enquiry, this time via Emanuel Swedenborg's vision of the spiritual, psychological and physical worlds. Swedenborg's teachings concerning divine influx and the laws of correspondence were central to Kent's understanding and practise of Hahnemannian homœopathy.

With the advent of the twentieth century, new paradigms burst upon the world scene. Sigmund Freud, again working from foundations already laid, revealed the world of instinctual drives and the consequences of their repression. His seminal work *The Interpretation of Dreams* was published in 1900.

Carl Jung, one-time pupil of Freud's, went far beyond the groundbreaking work of Freud. He revealed the mythological world with its gods, goddesses and sacred powers as still powerful and active in the collective unconscious. He again turned to the great visionaries of the past to find the language to describe the inner world that now opened before him. To Plato for the concept of archetypal powers. To the alchemists for their investigation of the symbolic world of the psyche. What he didn't know was that Hahnemann had, a century previously, been investigating, in provings, and in the context of the search for true healing agents, the dynamic reality that lies behind both psyche and soma. Hahnemann had, like the alchemists before him, been researching the properties of spirit in matter.

As the renewed investigation of the inner world emerged through the work of Jung (not really new, just a new twentieth century chapter in an investigation, a way of knowledge that had been developing for centuries, if not millennia) the invisible world within matter was also being revealed. Scientist like Niels Bohr and Albert Einstein were opening a door into the improbable world of the quantum field – the underlying reality lying within the mirage of matter. This again was a retelling of an old story. The sages of the East, through deep contemplation rather than scientific investigation, had gained profound insight into this world centuries before, calling it "void", "the unborn", "the tao", and so on.

Such is the world in which homœopathy finds itself today. Has much really changed? Have new discoveries really been made? Perhaps each new step in this voyage of discovery is more like a further unfolding or new view of a way of knowledge whose roots reach far back into history.

For Hahnemann the vital force is the dynamic movement that under-pins both mind and body. For us moderns it is also quantum field; it is instinct; it is symbol making as well as symptom forming.

This book is an attempt to speak the language of homœopathy in a world that has unprecedented knowledge of things ancient and modern – unprecedented awareness of unconscious drives, of mythology and archetypes, of the void and quantum field, and of what the alchemists were really up to in their efforts to transform base metal into gold.

Although homœopathy first appeared in the garb of nineteenth cen-tury empiricism, it really belongs to a timeless stream of thought and practice. It belongs to an ancient way, as well as to the modern world. We live in the postmodern world – post discovery of the unconscious, post quantum mechan-ical theory, post surrealist art. The practice and language of homœopathy must be recognisable to our world as well as honouring and embodying the Hahnemannian tradition and all that preceded it. This is evolution, not revo-lution. It is my hope that this book will be a contribution to that evolution.

Note to the reader
In some instances I have included additional information not immediately relevant to the main text. This additional text will be found with the relevant references at the end of the book.

Julian Carlyon
Stroud, Gloucestershire
June 2003

Chapter 1:
Wholeness and Symptoms

I want to begin with what the word "symptom" means to a homœopath. Our most immediate experience of disease is in the form of symptoms. Symptoms express disease and disintegration.

When we are healthy there is an absence of symptoms. Things feel, function and seem as they should. When health isn't present things don't seem right, feel right or function right. When health is absent there is distress, pain, disharmony or dysfunction in one part or another, to one extent or another.

A consideration of symptoms will also bring us to notions of wholeness and how wholeness gets lost, forgotten or undone. Health implies a functional and experiential wholeness. By this I mean a functional and experiential integration, in which the parts function harmoniously together as part of a greater whole. Things work in harmony; we feel in harmony; there is a sense of unity. However, it's also important to remember that integration is but the polarity of disintegration. The one leads to the other. Wholeness embraces both. As we shall see, it's the *identification* with one or the other that is problematic. Now, these ideas harbour far-reaching implications and considerations, which I'll attempt to unpack in the coming chapters.

So what we're going to do now, in the first few pages, is classify, briefly, the nature of symptoms – the signs and sensations that indicate the absence of wholeness. However, before doing that, I first want to say a bit more about the notion of wholeness. Because the notion of wholeness is so important, and because we'll return to it many times in the coming pages, I want to consider it a little here first. To do this I'm going to introduce the idea of holons. We'll look at holons and that will pave the way for a look at symptoms.

Holons

The term "holon" was originally coined by the philosopher Arthur Koestler.[1] The notion of holons has since been enthusiastically taken up by theorists such as the biologist Rupert Sheldrake and philosopher Ken Wilber. So, what are holons? Holons are the basic unit of creation.[2] Everything that comes into being is a holon. A holon is a self-organising whole, that is to say a whole that consists of parts that are organised into its wholeness. In turn a holon is part of a larger holon. Some examples. An atom is an organised whole of sub-atomic particles organised into a functioning whole. In turn atoms can be organised into greater wholes called molecules. A molecule is a self-organising whole which can be part of a larger self-organising whole called a cell, and so on. This is called a holarchy. It has been suggested that in the scheme of creation these holarchies have no limit, going to the infinitely small and infinitely large. We can apply this model to anything. For example the individual as a holon which is part of a society, which is part of a nation, which exists in the larger holon of the world, then solar system, thence galaxy and so on; or individual, within which there are smaller holons called organs and systems, thence cells, molecules, atoms and so on into the infinitely small. You get the idea. Even words and ideas are holons that exist in larger holons such as frames of reference, languages and so on.

Holons have a number of properties, a couple of which should be mentioned here. Firstly, because holons are self-organising wholes within larger self-organised wholes, they have two fundamental drives: on the one hand to protect and maintain their own integrity, and on the other to function as part of a larger community or holon. Secondly the growth, function and structure of a holon is maintained by an organising principle or organising field, which is called a morphic field or a vital field or a vital force.[3] All entities have such an organising field. It is the mind, memory and purpose of the entity.

Any holon also exists within a larger organising field, a larger holon. These larger fields are supra-ordinate fields, which hold and contain the parts in a higher, more embracing order and purpose.

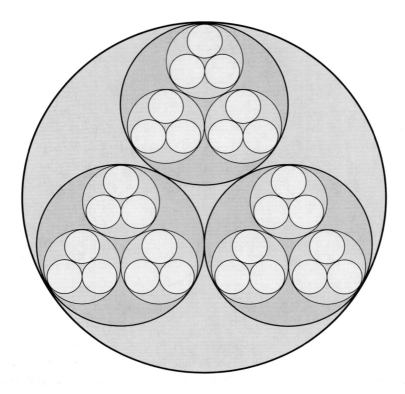

Fig. 1.1 Holons and holarchy

A holon contains smaller holons and is at the same time a part of a larger holon. For example a molecule is made up of smaller holons called atoms, and is at the same time part of a larger holon such as a cell. (After Rupert Sheldrake, *The Presence of the Past*)

Now we come to a property of holons that is particularly important for our understanding of symptoms. A holon has an inside and an outside. By this I mean that it has subjective consciousness and objective manifestation. On the one hand it has subjective experience, its own sense of itself and its world. On the other hand any holon can be seen from the outside. So there is the subjective experience of the holon (inside) on the one hand, and the objective view of the holon (outside) on the other.

Thus a holon can be known either from the inside or the outside. The inside is the subjective state of consciousness of the entity. This is its sense of itself and its experience of the world. Any form of consciousness, of whatever nature, belongs to the inner subjectivity of the holon. In the human being all

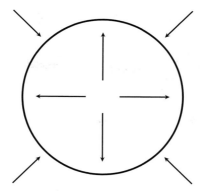

Fig. 1.2 Holon – inner and outer
The individual holon has subjective consciousness and can be objectively observed.

forms of sensation, feeling and perception belong to this class. (We can easily understand that a human being has consciousness. You know also that your dog has consciousness, a rather different form of consciousness to that of a human being, although there may be strong similarities! However it might be a little harder to grasp that a rock has consciousness – very, very different to the consciousness of a human being but, holon theory maintains, a form of consciousness nevertheless. From this point of view anything that exists, including such things as feelings, words, ideas, has some form of consciousness. Here are some examples of self-organising wholes which have their being within an organising field, or a field of "consciousness": atoms, minerals, cells, organs, plants, plant families, animals, animal classes (insects for example), human beings, human cultures, the Earth, planets, solar systems, galaxies, languages, ideas.)

The outside (of the holon) is what we can objectively know about something. This can be what it looks like, how it behaves and so on. We'll return to this inner and outer view in a while.

We can also look at how a holon relates to and is affected by the world around it. Thus there are four approaches to a holon – inner, outer, individual, communal. What's it like from the inside? What does it look like from the outside? How is it and what are its properties as an individual entity? How is it, and how does it behave as part of a larger whole or larger holon?

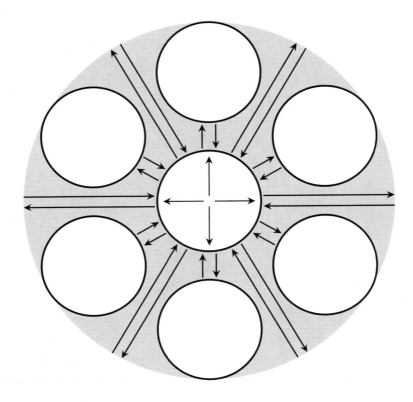

Fig. 1.3 Holon – individual and communal
The holon as part of a larger community, a larger holon.

Holon theory says that to have a comprehensive understanding of something one needs to know, if possible, what it's like from the inside, what its state of consciousness is like. One also needs to be able to observe it from the outside. Finally how is it as an individual and how is it as part of something larger (in other words how does it, as an individual, relate to and react to the world)?

Now, as far as the human individual goes, which is what concerns us here, holon theory is interesting and useful because it ties in with the way in which homœopaths have traditionally sought to classify and understand symptoms. Homœopathic theory has traditionally taught that a useful symptom, a comprehensive symptom, should have a sensation, a locality and a modality. In other words what are the internal sensations of disorder (sensation)? What are the localities and objective signs of dysfunction (locality)? How are these modified on the one hand by what a person does or doesn't do, and on the other, the influence of the world upon that person (modalities)?

In other words we must attempt to understand the inside of the person (the subjective world of the patient) as well as observe alterations in behaviour and function (objective view of the patient). We are also interested in how a person functions as part of the larger holons of family, society, culture and nature. This is revealed in the sensitivities and modalities.

Symptoms

We know when something is wrong because we have troubling sensations and things don't work as they should. This sense of things being wrong can be physical or psychological. We normally call the sensations and experiences of things being wrong, symptoms.

Homœopaths see symptoms as the most valuable guide to the selection of a homœopathic remedy. When the life of mind or body is disturbed or dysfunctional, this disturbance or dysfunction reveals itself in symptoms.[4]

Homœopaths see symptoms in terms of sensation, function and modality.

The word "sensation", in its usage here, refers to the whole domain of subjective experience, both in mind and body, of ourselves and our world. This is the inner domain of health and disease. Function, on the other hand, relates to the objective data. Which organ or area of the body is affected and what is the objective evidence of dysfunction? How has the appearance or behaviour of a person altered?

Sensation is the inner experience of a problem (the inside of the holon). This could be psychological, a distressing feeling such as sadness for example. It could be physical, pain or discomfort in a part of the body.

Disturbed function, on the other hand, is the outer evidence of the problem. Discharges or inflammation are typical signs of disturbed function. Even inflammation of inner organs that can only be seen by extensions of the eye such as X-ray apparatus, still belong to the "outer", objective view of things. For example a person could have inflammation of the colon (objective, locality), accompanied by burning pain (sensation), which is worse for movement (modality).

When someone is experiencing fear (sensation, subjective) this can be apparent in the way they behave, move, speak and so on (objective signs).

Modalities (we'll come to them more fully in a minute) refer to what a person does or doesn't do to avoid pain (and maximise pleasure) and to the way they are affected for better or worse by the environment. Thus we have a complete circle of symptoms offering an all-round understanding of the human holon. Inner (sensation), outer (function), individual (do's and don'ts) and collective (effect of the world at large).

So with the help of homœopathic theory (aided by holon theory) we can see that to understand a person in sickness, and indeed in health, it is necessary to have a complete view. What is the inner state of the person? What is the outer state of the person? What do they do about it? How are they affected by the world at large? We can see that homœopaths have traditionally sought to obtain this all-round view. Of course this all-round view is an ideal which can usually only be approximated in practice. A person's case history usually has more of the subjective, or more of the objective, or has stronger modalities. Also the emphasis may be more on the physical or psychological level. Nevertheless the homœopath seeks to gather this all-round view of the patient in the knowledge that one facet or another could provide the vital clue that unlocks the understanding of the whole.

It's also important to remember that the subjective and the objective are two views of the same state of being. They are not different. The feelings and perceptions that a person has are the inner experience of their state of being. The dysfunctions (physical and psychological) and modes of behaviour that can be observed are the same state of being, now seen from the outside.

Modalities highlight the sensitivities and needs of that person's state of being in relation to the surrounding world.

When the homœopath attempts to understand a patient it is best if he can grasp the inner state of the person, the changes in function and behaviour, and the modalities, as a single whole. Even when some of this information is lacking it is possible to get an insight into the whole when we remember that outer symptoms reflect the same state of being (or suffering) as do even the deepest inner sensations. Thus the behaviour, gestures and apparent symptoms of a person can be revealing of a person's inner state. We'll return to this important point later.

Pain

People seek help from a homœopath because they are suffering. They are experiencing some form of pain or disquiet in mind, body, or both. This can range from mild discomfort to agony. Pain can be physical or emotional. Physical pain includes every imaginable painful sensation coming from inside or outside the body. We know emotional pain as grief, sadness, anger, fear and so on. Some kinds of inner pain, like the pain of being denied personal, political or religious rights we might call mental or spiritual pain.

Pain is a troublesome sensation. It interrupts the flow of life and consciousness. Any troublesome sensation, any awareness that troubles us, whether it be in the mind or body, is, in the homœopathic view of things, a symptom. But let's get one thing straight here. We are not saying that symptoms are bad, or that pain is bad. That of course is not the same as saying we would not like, sometimes more than anything in the world, to get rid of pain. What we are saying here is that pain expresses a state of disorder. Symptoms of pain or dysfunction mean that something somewhere within us is struggling or out of balance. This means that something within us needs to change or is trying to change. We all experience pain as something out of the ordinary. It draws and focuses our attention. It reminds us of our presence, or it reminds us of a part of ourselves. Pain of any kind, in the soul or body, pulls awareness into ourselves. Whether we like it or not it makes us self-aware. We'll come back later to the connection between pain and awareness.

There is an additional consideration here, which is this. A person may not be able to communicate about certain aspects of their inner experience or their inner condition, for one simple reason. The experience or sensation, because it is painful or felt as unpleasant or unacceptable is repressed. It does not surface into the individual's awareness, and thus they are unable to tell us about it directly.

A troubling sensation or disturbance of function in the body, which alerts us that all is not well, may be suppressed by medical intervention. Thus the expression of the disease is denied.

When it comes to psychological pain the dynamics of suppression are subtler and more deeply rooted. This is because we learn to block out what troubles us. We repress what we find difficult and painful. In the coming chapters we'll need to consider the connection between the suppression of pain

– the suppression of what we feel or judge to be painful, bad or unacceptable

– and the dynamics of disease.

Modalities

So, in homœopathy we need to understand the human condition from the inside and the outside. We listen to a person's description of their experience of body and mind. We also listen to their description of their experience of the world, their worldly experience. We also note alterations in physical function and psychological behaviour. We also need to consider (in accordance with holon theory) the relationship a person has with their internal world on the one hand and with the world of which they are a part on the other. In other words how are individuals affected by their own nature, the world of nature around them and the human world of society and culture? This brings us to modalities.

The notion of modalities embraces everything that a person does or doesn't do in order to feel good and avoid feeling bad. People generally seek what makes them feel better and avoid what makes them feel worse. This is because people seek to maintain a sense of inner equilibrium, control, autonomy and comfort. A person tries to maintain the psychological and physical conditions for feeling OK. We naturally try to avoid or minimise physical pain. Psychologically we like to avoid pain and minimise conflict. Thus a person exerts their will, often unconsciously, to try and control the world in and around them. Here are some examples of things that people do or avoid in order to feel better. Physically – lying, standing, adopting certain positions and movements, keeping still, moving, eating, fasting, eating certain foods, avoiding certain foods, staying indoors, opening the windows. Psychologically – seeking company, avoiding company, controlling others, controlling oneself.

Under the heading of modalities we must also include the way a person is affected by the world within them. We are subject to all kinds of instinctive and involuntary processes within. These include the functions of the body, such as breathing, digestion and the menstrual cycle. As well as this must be included our instincts such as sexual response and self-preservation. We must include loves and hates. We must include all kinds of impulses and the movements of the heart. We must consider all that we are moved by and the powerful motives that stir within our own depths. In this inner world we find powers of nature in much the same way as we find powers of nature in the external world. We can find a harmony with these powers, but not control them. The attempt to control or subjugate our own nature leads, as we will see, to all kinds of trouble. It was not without good reason that Jung referred to the unconscious psyche – the world of inner nature and inner powers – as the "objective psyche." [5] In other words, it is as objectively real and true to its own laws as the external world of nature.

We are also subject to the external world of nature. We are influenced, for better or worse, and whether we like it or not, by climate, weather, season; by the rhythms of night and day, and those of moon, sun, planets and beyond.

We are also influenced by the human world. We are subject to the influence of people in a number of ways. For example it is now known how profound the influence of family, parents and siblings is in the formation of a person's character and responses. Beyond this the family itself is subject to social, cultural and religious conditions.

We should also contemplate the relationship we have with and the way we are moved by the numinous (the spiritual, the divine, by whatever name we know it). Desires and aversions in the end are rooted in the deepest desires for love, connection and spiritual well-being. A holistic therapy must realise that this is so and take it into account; otherwise, it would not be addressing the deepest causes of health and sickness in the human being.

In this opening chapter I have attempted to lay a foundation by clarifying the nature of symptoms. We're now ready to go further and ask how a lack of wholeness with its accompanying sense of "dis-ease" comes about.

Chapter 2

Cycle and Polarity

In the first chapter we considered health and sickness in terms of immediate experience – how people experience themselves and the world, and the way in which this is altered in the conditions that we call illness or disease. In this chapter, in a more philosophical approach, I want to turn our attention to the characteristics of human constitution, which give rise to a fundamental disposition to sickness and disease. I want to do this so that our understanding of illness and of the homœopathic approach to healing flows from an understanding of first causes in human constitution. In doing this I am following a path already trodden by homœopathic physician philosophers of the past, who have put at the centre of their medical philosophies an understanding of original dispositions to suffering, with the intention that this should guide the practical work of homœopathic therapy.

First let's consider how we're made. Let's consider constitution. We can say firstly there are two fundamental aspects of constitution. These we can call nature and consciousness. However, I want to emphasise that these two aspects are in the end only two faces of one being. In truth there is one being, one consciousness. This being is present in human constitution as both nature and consciousness. These two can appear different, but are in fact one.

That said, let's take nature first. Hahnemann used the term "vital force" to describe the presence and activity of nature in human constitution. He tells us that the vital force is "spirit like." In a more modern idiom Edward Whitmont speaks of it as an "information field." [1] These are important and helpful concepts, but are nevertheless not our immediate experience of the *life* of the life force. Rather the presence of life is my flesh, bone and pulsation of blood. It is in fleeting sensation as well as searing physical pain. It is in gut feeling, emotional turmoil or the subtle, often unacknowledged feelings that are my navigator in the stream of life. The vital force is the sensitivity and responsiveness of life coursing through our veins.

All of this is the presence and movement of nature within us. It is a dynamic presence that is rhythmic and cyclical. The oldest symbol of our vital, changing, seasonal being is the circle. The circle symbolises both containment and circular – or cyclical – movement. This suggests that each person and each creature is a self-contained and self-maintaining whole that is at the same time in rhythmic interplay and intimate exchange with surrounding life. You are eating and breathing the world, laughing and crying as the world flows through you.

The turning of the circle represents the way of nature. All of nature is cyclical – cycles of respiration, inspiration and expiration, of eating and defecation, of light and dark, of birth and death; the cycles of day, month and year; of sun, moon and planets; the turning of the galaxy itself.

Human nature partakes in all this. Indeed this is the weave of your physicality. You, in your vital presence, pulse to your own rhythm, which at the same time is the rhythm of nature. Beating heart, inflow and outflow of breath, peristaltic rhythm of digestion and electrical flash of nerve and synapse. We breathe in and out with winter and summer, day and night. This is the rhythm of life from the moment we gasp our first breath to the time we step through the portal of life's greatest mystery.

The circle represents movements and relationships within you – of physical systems, of feelings and thoughts – as well as the cycles of interchange with the surrounding world – liquids, nutrients, air, sensations, feelings, and so on. All of this constitutes the activity of the vital force.

The circle also represents enclosed form. The vital force is responsible for form as well as for function. There is something that, amidst the activity and cyclical change of mind and body, ensures that you are still you. There is something which holds the pattern of a person's unique shape and character, despite the fact that what a person is made of – oxygen, water, nutrients, mineral salts, as well as feelings, intuitions, thoughts – is in a constant state of cycle, change and flux.

A human life is marked by it highs and lows, its day and night and seasons. And it is through just such a journey that we become etched and shaped. Through seasoning, richness and flavour of character is revealed. Something in us endures and deepens while every single aspect of what's inside and outside lives and dies according to the law of its being.

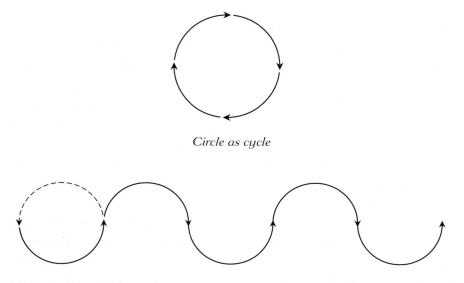

Circle as cycle

Circle as wave: the motion of the circle spread out through time.

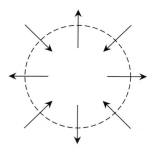

Circle as enclosed form in rhythmic exchange with its environment.

Fig. 2.1 Circle as cycle, wave and form

The solar self

Lets turn our consideration now to the part of ourselves that doesn't seem to belong to the vital rhythm of earthly life. There is something in us that is quite different from our earthly nature. Humans have an ability and a need to throw light on things. The philosophers of the past, who recognised the correspondence between things, said that this is like the presence of the Sun in our constitution. In the Greek pantheon this was the domain of Apollo, god of light; god of the arts, prophecy, archery, law-giving and medicine – in short he was a god of culture, order and rationality. This is the principle of human consciousness. It gives us the ability to know the world: to name things, to understand ourselves, to understand things, and to use things. This gives human beings, to a far greater degree than any other of the Earth's creatures, the ability to look after themselves and the world. It gives us the ability to take note of the past and make provision for the future (prophesy). It makes humans very successful and adaptable creatures. It was meant to be thus, but there was a price to pay.

The principle of consciousness bestows the ability to bring things into the light of day. The development of consciousness meant that humans learnt to see more clearly. But we all know that light casts a shadow and creates a world of light and dark. Humans learnt to discriminate. This word comes from the Latin *discriminare,* meaning to divide. The property of the light of the Sun in human makeup gives us the ability to discern (from Latin *cernere,* to separate). We know and understand by separating things one from another, and by separating ourselves from the world. Thus the gift of consciousness also creates division and separation.

It is interesting here to look at other words relating to discriminate; words like crime and criminal for example. This relationship of words can be very revealing. The acquisition of discriminating consciousness by human beings is often depicted in mythology as a crime against the gods, a crime that must be punished. In the Greek story of Prometheus, who stole fire from Olympus to give to human beings, this crime – a crime from the point of view of the gods, but the heroic act of a saviour from humanity's point of view – leads, as a consequence of the wrath of Zeus at the audacity of Prometheus, to the sicknesses of human kind and the necessity to acquire healing powers.

The development of this discriminating ability meant a rift in nature. Humans, although part of nature, in the act of acquiring the ability to think and reflect, stood aside from nature. They stood aside from themselves and their world and this inevitably meant a rift in human makeup and a break in the wholeness of nature.

I am not here going to attempt to place this event – the advent of human consciousness – in a historical context. I am instead alluding to a tendency that may have emerged over millions of years, through man's many developments – walking upright, as a tool user, as inventor of fire, as inventor of art and ritual, as inventor of language, as farmer, city dweller and so on. The important point in our consideration of health and disease is that this discriminating consciousness – this light-giver and light-bearer – progressively lost its connection with the world of nature. It became a usurper on the world stage. This part of ourselves decided that since it was like the Sun, it also should become eternal and unchanging.[2] It should stand outside the round of earthly life and death. This means that there is something in our makeup, and has been for a very long time, that doesn't want to die, that wants to rise above the round of life, to conquer death.

However all life on Earth is cyclical and rhythmic. Above all it lives and dies. You cannot have an earthly life and avoid this fundamental truth. It is a truth that rules everything human – our bodies, feelings, relationships, thoughts, ideas, cultures and civilisations. Thus it has been said that to know how to live in this world is, above all, to know how to die.

In mythological traditions the break in nature that results from the presence of discriminating consciousness has often been understood as a kind of wound.[3] Human beings in the course of their development have sustained a deep wound to their nature. They have also wounded the earth.

For many thousands of years the healing of this wound was the central concern of culture, art and healing practices. For thousands of years, ever since man began to reflect, there were those amongst the people charged with knowing and understanding this inevitable wound in human nature and the life of the world. The shamans and sages of the past understood that the presence of human consciousness, seated in the divided cerebral hemispheres, meant a split in the world. These wise ones and medicine men and women also understood that as long as ritual practises, which reminded people of their place and belonging in the whole, were maintained, then the wound to human and worldly nature might be closed. The advent of human consciousness meant that the compact with the whole had to be continually remade. This was to be done in the seasonal ceremonials during which the gods, the powers that preside in heaven, on Earth, and in human nature, were honoured. The giving of medicine and the interpretation of dreams was also carried out with reference to this greater picture.[4] Humans are part of nature and the cosmos. It was understood that things would be well if the life, rhythm and order of nature and cosmos was maintained, despite the splitting of human consciousness from nature and within itself. The intention was to offset the dangers of the gift of human consciousness.

Nature, discrimination and reality

We are saying, then, that there are two fundamental dimensions to our makeup (although, as we've said, this apparent duality is in reality one). These are the life of nature on the one hand and the presence of consciousness on the other. As consciousness emerges out of nature, during the course of human evolution, it acquires the capacity to discriminate. In doing this it acquires the ability to judge and to choose. Put very simply, consciousness can now choose between what it perceives to be good and what it perceives to be bad. Thus we can see that the rhythm and cycle of nature is superseded by a form of consciousness that tends to polarity, and which thus carries within it the seeds of conflict and opposition.

There is however another important point here. Nature and discriminating mind are not the whole story, far from it.

According to the philosophy of the Upanishads, both nature and discriminating mind spring from the one source, the unmanifest, the divine ground of all manifestation. At this transpersonal level (the source, the ground, the unmanifest) all sense of separation is overcome. All sense of separation is understood as illusion. There is only oneness, only divine unity.

The discriminating mind is incapable of knowing and experiencing this higher reality. It can only divide. However, there is a higher mind, the buddhi mind, which is the pure intelligence capable of opening us to the true source of being.[5] Pure mind is fully present, spacious and free of the illusions of past, future and separateness.

The evolution of consciousness

I think it would be helpful now to introduce the notion of the development of human consciousness and its place in the scheme of things. In very general terms we can say that there are three phases in the development of human consciousness. These can be broadly categorised as unconsciousness, self-consciousness and transpersonal consciousness. Transpersonal consciousness is sometimes referred to as higher consciousness, transcendent consciousness, integrative consciousness or super consciousness (see Chapter 3). These phases unfold in the collective development of the human species as well as in the development of the human individual.

Thus there is a pathway, in the life of an individual as well as in the life of the species, from unconsciousness, through the development of self-consciousness, to transpersonal consciousness. This entails a movement from unconscious wholeness to a consciousness of self that is accompanied by a splitting and fragmentation of wholeness, to conscious reintegration and wholeness.[6] Unconscious wholeness, fragmentation, conscious wholeness.

This is the big developmental story playing itself out through human history and through the lives – probably many, many lives – of individuals. The collective story and the individual story are the big version and the small version of the same story. We'll look briefly at them both.

Collective development

In the great sweep of human evolution these stages (unconsciousness, self consciousness and super consciousness) can be thought of as corresponding to the distant past, the historical period (which we can loosely call the present), and the future of human evolution. So, past, present and future; unconsciousness, self-consciousness, transcendent consciousness. (I should emphasise that these terms are of course relative. In this context unconsciousness does not mean an absence of consciousness. All of nature is alive, and in one way or another conscious. It means that there is a relative absence of an awareness of self. In the animal world a deer has more sense of self than a worm. However the sense of self in a deer is not as clear and differentiated as it is in a human. The deer lives its life in the wholeness of the embrace of nature to a greater degree than a human. The important point is that these terms are relative. More or less unconscious relative to other stages of development or other species. More or less self-conscious. More or less conscious wholeness.)

Human self-consciousness originally appears out of the matrix of nature in the prehistoric era. No date can be put on this, although it is likely that its gradual development is reflected through key transitional stages such as walking erect, using tools, discovery of fire, evidence of ritual, the appearance of art, and so on.[7]

As far as recent evolutionary history goes it is generally recognised (within orthodox views of evolution and history anyway) that modern man, homo sapiens, the species that knows that he is conscious, appeared about fifty thousand years ago. More recently still the whole notion of individuality and individual responsibility as a dominant cultural ideal seems to have come dramatically to the fore about three thousand five hundred years ago.[8] In this latter period we witness the emergence of heroes and saviours in mythology. In the iron age we see the emergence of war as an ideal and the praise of conquest. This is really the beginning of our own era, in which conquest and power became the dominant gods. Nature and natural life becomes something to be controlled. Thus the emergence of the ideal of the self-conscious personality begins to disrupt the life of the earth. As this process gathers momentum in the last three or four thousand years individuals develop a stronger and more enduring sense of self which is concomitant to a greater capacity to disrupt there own natural being.

In the past, on the other hand, during the prehistoric era, mythologies celebrated the life giving presence of the great goddess – mythologies in which the wholeness of the Earth and nature was held sacred. There was wholeness, but probably little sense of individual freedom. In fact individuality and difference may have been seen as dangerous and undesirable.[9] Of course individuality is still frequently treated with suspicion today.

What about the future? The next stage of human evolution asks for conscious reintegration. This means that our higher capacities are to be used to heal ourselves, society and the Earth. The next stage of human evolution requires that individuals work in conscious co-operation with their own nature, with each other and with the Earth. This constitutes the consciously synthesising phase of cultural development. If this era were to fail to develop, the prospects for the race would be very bleak. In fact I believe the race would be a spent force that would eventually descend into terminal decline.

Individual Development

Individual development follows a similar path, which I will only mention here in brief outline because we'll look at it in more detail in the next chapter. In utero and the early weeks of infancy the infant is in symbiosis with the mother. There is little, if any, sense of differentiation from the mother. As the months and years go by the conscious individual, characterised by a sense of self, emerges by stages towards the goal of the integrated individual. If this unfolding towards a mature individual is successful then the way is open for the emergence of capacities of consciousness, love, wisdom and freedom, which are characteristic of integrated and transpersonal states of being. In this view of things these higher stages of development can only emerge success-fully on the basis of healthy self-development. In history these higher stages of development have only been achieved by a very few. At the beginning of the twenty-first century more individuals stand at the threshold of these more embracing states of being.

Having given this brief overview of consciousness we'll return to the subject at hand. In the rest of this chapter, and indeed in the book, we will attempt to understand how the rhythm of life becomes stuck and fixed into patterns of disease as a result of the presence of human self-consciousness. Once human self-consciousness has appeared in the world, causing a funda-mental and unhealing wound in life's fabric, then the vital force can no longer restore order on its own without the aid of the once and always healing art.

Opposites

The life of body and soul on Earth is characterised by cycle and rhythm. The presence of self-consciousness introduces the dynamics of polarity. However because there are differences and tensions within the kingdom of the human soul, there need not necessarily be conflict to the point of warfare and disintegration. The ancient Chinese symbol of yin and yang is a profound and elegant image of the relationship of opposites. It shows yang and yin, male and female, light and dark, engaged in a serpentine dance, in which one coils into the other – the one bearing the seed of the other as it reaches its maximum potential and moves into decline. It is a symbol of the dance of opposites, imagined as a sensuous "erotic" pairing. It suggests the harmonious and cyclical flow of opposites. The ancient Chinese philosophers particularly understood the cyclical nature of events, where things turn into their opposite through cyclical flow. They studied these laws of nature, and introduced cultural practices in an attempt to harmonise human activity with them.

The cross is another archetypal symbol of the relationships between opposites. As a symbol it can be read in a number of ways. It stands for the interpenetration of the earthly world and the archetypal world. It shows heaven above and the underworld below. It also stands for the four directions, the four seasons and the four elements. As a symbol of human consciousness it reveals the nature of our discriminating consciousness. This consciousness works through comparison and thus brings about the possibility of conflicting opposites. Through this form of consciousness we learn to choose. We learn to accept and reject. It is through this consciousness that we are able to acquire learnt ideas about what is good and what is bad, and to choose on that basis.

Discriminating consciousness also gives us the capacity to make judgements about ourselves. Our need to belong means that we learn, very early in life, to make judgements about good and bad, right and wrong, and so on. We couldn't become self-aware human beings without going through this process.

However, this capacity to judge almost always means that we learn to accept certain sides of ourselves (labelled the good) and reject other sides of ourselves (labelled the bad).

In the course of time the opposites in our nature (what we feel to be good, what we feel to be bad) may become enemies. These opposites may both clamour for attention. The individual may be riven by internal conflicts. Or worse, the opposites may become so dissociated that psychic integrity breaks down to the point of psychosis and psychopathic behaviour.

At any rate we often struggle to deal with conflicting needs or try to hold together apparently opposing parts of our own nature. Disease, it can be said, arises from conflicts within ourselves that we are unable to contain or which in some way fragment us.

The symbol of the cross is not all bad news. Far from it. The good news is that it has a centre (sometimes enclosed in a circle) where opposites meet. The symbol of the cross tells us there is a centre where opposites can be re-solved. Thus out of conflict there emerges the possibility of a more accepting and embracing consciousness. New possibilities arise out of pain and disinte-gration. In a sense becoming healthy means developing the art of being in the still centre whilst knowing and accepting the opposites within oneself.

The marriage of opposites

In the symbolism of cultures such as the native American and the Celtic cross is often shown in a circle. Thus in the symbol of the cross in the circle the opposites are contained within the embrace of wholeness. The womb of space contains us, and the serpent of time turns within us and around us. The opposites of winter and summer, of above and below are simply part of the pulse of time and space.

This symbol suggests that it is possible for our choosing nature to work in harmony with our rhythmic nature. It suggests that all the abilities that humans

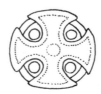

have acquired as a result of the presence of discriminating consciousness can be put at the service of the wholeness and power of the feminine presence, which is embodied in the Earth and the life of nature.

Consciousness has evolved out of nature. Nature gave birth to human consciousness because she needs its presence. In the mythologies of the past this event was depicted as a goddess who gives birth to a divine child, a hero or saviour.[10] For example, it is Isis who gives birth to Osiris, her son and lover. There is a need for human consciousness in the world. However, the purpose of this consciousness is to co-operate with nature. The purpose is to become a light within nature. What we have seen is that human self-consciousness has attempted to acquire power over nature. This process – the attempt to acquire power over nature – occurs in the development of culture and in the development of the individual. In a culture this makes possible the violation of nature. In an individual it makes possible the repression, denial or distortion of one's own nature. It is this possibility, so I maintain, that forms the foundation of human chronic sickness.

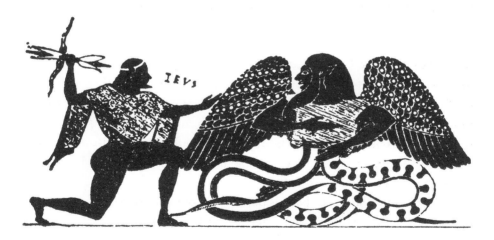

Fig. 2.2 Hero and serpent (Zeus and Typhon)
The motif of the battle between hero (or god) and serpent or dragon is a potent mythological theme. Psychologists such as Jung have seen the motif as a symbol of the struggle of self-consciousness to free itself from unconsciousness. The motif also suggests the domination of the natural by heroic self-consciousness.

The nineteenth century pioneer of American homœopathy, James Tyler Kent, also spoke of these matters. He maintained that disease is a result of wrong willing, which in turn arises from wrong thinking.[11] I understand him to mean that this is what happens when the human individual identity that we have been discussing becomes separated from nature and takes willing unto itself. Thence human identity becomes dislocated from its natural roots, and the notion of free will, without any reference to the order, rhythm and season of life on Earth, holds sway. As we have seen, the emergence of human self-consciousness with its concomitant sense of difference and separation has been a necessary and desirable part of human evolution. It has brought many gifts such as the ability to reflect, prophecy and the arts. At the same time it has produced a tragic wounding of the wholeness of nature both within us and in the life of the Earth. I believe that Hahnemann also alludes to this state of affairs when he writes "the ... life force ... was only instilled in our organism to continue our life on a harmonious course as long as the organism is healthy, *but not to cure itself in diseases* [italics mine]." [12] In other words, as long as the wholeness of nature existed – for billions of years before human consciousness entered the scene – the vital force, that is the instinctual mind, artistry and memory of nature held unchallenged sovereignty.

Healing

For any meaningful healing to come about this wound must be addressed. There must be a healing of the rift between consciousness and nature, between above and below, and between male and female. Let's finish this chapter by looking at two symbols that point to this possibility.

The staff of Asclepius

A variation on the symbol of cross and circle is the healing staff of Asclepius. Asclepius is the god of healing credited by the ancient Greeks with the invention of medicine. It is an image of particular importance to homœopaths. The symbol pictures

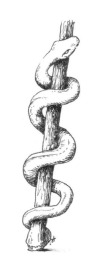

Fig. 2.3 Staff of Asclepius

a serpent twined around a staff. It is a variation on the image of circle and cross, showing the rhythmic life force, represented as a serpent, drawn up upon the structure of the staff. It shows the rod of conscious thought and wilful action embraced by the serpent of rhythmic life. The image suggests that healing involves the marriage of these two and even suggests the coupling of lingam and yoni in a sacred marriage.

The Heart

When we look at the heart we see its likeness to the symbol of the cross in the circle. Four chambers, four elements, above and below, left and right; all this meets in the heart. There are other kinds of meetings in the heart as well. Active and passive, male and female, meet in the heart in the exchange between arterial and venous blood (working together with the pulmonary circulation). High and low also meet in the heart in that the heart has two systems, one supplying the lungs and one the rest of the body. The heart is also the centre of exchange between inner and outer in that it pumps the oxygen and nutrients received from the external world around the body and draws the returning venous blood to itself.

Thus many opposites meet in the heart – male and female, left and right, above and below, inner and outer. Thus it is in the heart that the opposites can meet and combine in the pulse and rhythmic exchange of life. Here a person may find the union of male and female, above and below, and inner and outer. The marriage of consciousness and nature takes place in the heart. It is the embodiment of this marriage in the human being. The heart is the natural centre of human constitution, and it is through the heart that we belong to the world. In fact if you take the "h" at the end of "Earth", and move it to the front you have the word "heart".

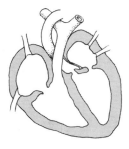 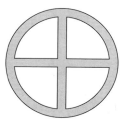

In this chapter we have attempted to understand the twin processes of the emergence of self-consciousness, with its innate polarising tendency, and the wounding of the wholeness of nature. We have seen how inextricably these two are intertwined. I have suggested that disease arises out of this wound. In the next chapter we'll consider individual development and the way in which disease appears in the individual.

Chapter 3:
Self and Shadow

In the last chapter we took a general overview of the human condition. Now I want to get more specific. I want to look at individual development from birth. In doing so we'll attempt to understand the genesis, pattern and process of individual sickness.

Before doing that however it would be a good idea to contemplate how things might be before conception and birth. Although this is an area that is beyond everyday knowledge, it is something that is widely spoken of in various spiritual traditions. Here I'm going to draw on an account given by Plato. It is a poetic account. In appealing to the imagination it offers an approach to a domain of reality that lies beyond the reach of ordinary consciousness.

Plato says that your soul chooses its incarnation. Put another way, something deep within you chooses your destiny. This word "destiny" is from the Latin, *destino*, meaning that which is woven or fixed with chords and threads.[1] In other words it is something you cannot escape from, even though you might struggle against it. According to Plato it is the Goddess Necessity, she who turns the spindle upon which is wound the fabric of our lives, who presides over this choice of destiny. It is the need to become more deeply ourselves that attracts us to, indeed necessitates, our destiny. According to this story, the soul passes before the three fates, daughters of Necessity. Lachesis measures the fabric of destiny; she apportions the soul's destiny. Clotho spins the fabric. Atropos cuts life's thread; she makes the chosen lot irreversible.[2]

However before the soul clothes itself in the weave of events, people and ideas that it has chosen – a woven pattern or design, not of mechanically fixed events, but, in the language of quantum physics, of probabilities – it passes beneath the throne of Necessity and thence through the stifling heat of the plain of Leith, the plain of oblivion and forgetfulness. It is here also that the soul drinks from the River of Neglectfulness, whose waters no vessel can hold. Thus the soul forgets and neglects its destiny.[3] It is as though at birth a person falls into a deep sleep, forgetting who they are and why they are here – a condition that is then often reinforced through education and upbringing. From this point of view life is a search, often unconscious, for what has been forgotten, what is felt to be lost. It is this search that draws us into the highways and byways of life. Becoming whole means, as it were, coming to your senses, remembering who you really are and the reason you chose to be here.

Stages of development

We have seen that the soul's lot on Earth amounts, in broad terms, to a developmental journey from unconsciousness, through the development of a self conscious "I", to an eventual reunion with the divine wholeness out of which self-conscious individuality emerged in the first place. I want now to look a little more closely at the stages of development of the self conscious "I". As the unfolding of the individual takes place the self must pass through key stages of development. Health depends on the healthy establishment and unfolding of these stages. Problems or traumas can occur at any stage. When these problems or traumas remain unresolved they form the foundations on which chronic disease can develop. I'll attempt to show you in this chapter the important implications this has for homœopathic understanding and practice.

Developmental psychology theory contains a large body of careful and painstaking research. The stages of development through which an individual grows and develops have been observed and documented with the rigour of the best scientific investigation. I am going to introduce you to a developmental model based on the work of Ken Wilber.[4] He himself is not a clinician, but a philosopher and transpersonal psychology theorist. In his work he has analysed the findings of leading clinicians and researchers in the field of developmental psychology. He has found much commonality in these findings, and on this basis has created a synthesis. I have taken the map that he has proposed of the fundamental stages of human self-conscious development as the basis for the material of this chapter. His developmental map is based largely on the work of leading researchers such as Jean Piaget, Margaret Mahler, Abraham Maslow, Lawrence Kohlberg, Freud, Jung, and many others. As well as this he has mapped the higher reaches of transpersonal or spiritual consciousness, drawing on the many wisdom traditions of the world that have described these non-personal modes of consciousness.

He has suggested a seven-stage model of the development of the integrated human being. He then goes on to describe four further stages of transpersonal consciousness.

I'll name these stages now, before going on to discuss them in a little more detail. The first stage is referred to as zero (because the whole is here still relatively intact). This sequence of seven is then followed by the four stages of transpersonal consciousness, which we also will touch on later. Given below are the stages of development of self-consciousness based on Wilber's synthesis of the theoretical models of leading researchers in the field.

0. Intrauterine/birth
1. Physical/physiocentric
2. Emotional
3. Mental/conceptual
4. Rule/role mind
5. Formal-reflexive awareness
6. Vision-logic

The map charts the emergence and differentiation of self-consciousness. This emergence takes place by stages. At each stage of development the basic structure of consciousness corresponding to that stage is established. In other words a sense of physical self is established, followed by a sense of emotional self hood, followed by a sense of mental selfhood, and so on. Each mode of being should then develop and adapt throughout the remainder of the individual's life.

Phases of the stages

Each stage consists of three phases. In the first phase the self has to rise to the challenge of growing into the new stage. In the second phase the self establishes itself at the new stage of development. In this phase the self begins to differentiate itself from the reality characteristic of that stage of development. In the third phase the identification with that stage of development breaks up, initiating the necessity for the self to grow and move on to the more embracing form of consciousness offered by the next stage of development.

Only when the self begins to realise that it is different from a particular level of reality can it become a differentiated self that is able to respond to, learn from and act upon the dynamics of that particular level of being. Only when it has successfully done this can it move on to the next stage. For example, in utero and in the first weeks of life the infant is in a more or less complete symbiotic oneness with the mother. Any sense of presence is more or less completely united with the presence of the mother. In the first few weeks of life the infant begins to realise that its physical body is separate from the environment. The differentiation of a physical sense of self starts to take place. However at this stage (physical) the self is still identified with the emotional environment. The emotional self has not yet differentiated. At the start of the emotional stage, although a sense of physical presence has begun to emerge, the infant is still a bundle of feelings and emotions in complete identification with its emotional environment. There is as yet little sense of an emotional self. The infant has little sense of itself as a separate emotional entity, and therefore little sense that its feelings might be different from another. In the second phase of the emotional stage the self begins to realise that it is a self with feelings. It begins to realise that feelings are *happening to it,* either from inside or outside. In this sense it begins to differentiate from the feeling world. Previous to this "awakening" it had been identified with the feeling level, responding to the currents of feeling within and around it without particular awareness of its own selfhood within these currents. In the final phase of the emergence of the emotional sense of self, consciousness is preparing for, or resisting, the necessity to be "born" into the next stage of the emergence of self-consciousness, the mental/conceptual stage.

Each stage has this beginning, middle and end structure. Each round in the emergence of self-consciousness sees the self at first identified with a particular level (the emotional for example), then established as a self at that level (a self that *has* feelings and emotions), and then beginning to dis-identify with that level in order that it may be "born" into the next level. The emotional self, for example, cannot continue to be *only* an emotional self. It has to grow beyond the self-centredness of emotions and learn to engage with the world through thought and concept. It has to give up its existence as *only* emotional, and be born into the wider possibilities of awareness and communication characteristic of the mental/conceptual level. The self can be born here into a wider world that transcends the narcissism of emotional existence.

Stages of development (continued)

As each stage of development is encountered, the self should, in Wilber's words, "transcend and include." Each stage emerges out of the previous stage as the chick out of the egg. The new consciousness – and this will turn out to be a fundamentally important point – should include, rather than deny or repress, the previous stage. For example if the mental self emerges at the expense of the well-being of the emotional self, dysfunction will result. For healthy development to take place each level needs to be a stable foundation for the next stage of growth. There needs to be integration of what has gone before.

Each stage of development offers new opportunities for growth and awareness. However as the self emerges there is also the potential for accompanying anxiety, conflict and pathology. Conflict may emerge at any stage. Trauma may be sustained at any stage. When this happens parts of the self can get stuck at previous stages of development. There is dissociation rather than integration within the psychophysical system of the individual. Parts of the self can get split off. These parts of the self, in some way traumatised or wounded, are unable to grow and develop healthily. They remain as sources of difficulty and conflict in the subconscious psyche. Such "problems" can get buried by the necessities of the next stage of development, becoming subterranean wounds that hamper subsequent stages of unfolding. The emerging self simply represses areas of pain, conflict and difficulty that are encountered on life's path. Emotional trauma or conflict, for example, will be driven underground as the mental/conceptual self rises to the challenge of conceptual thinking and education.

An infant might experience difficulty in the first few weeks of life, just as physical self-consciousness is emerging. This could be a sense that the mother is not reliably present. Maybe the mother doesn't feed the child when it cries with hunger. Perhaps the child experienced a physical shock or a severe fright. In the very worst cases the child could be abused. As such a person goes through life they will carry the feeling of the unsafe or traumatised infant. This is a split off part of themselves that remains infantile, undeveloped, troublesome, and in need of healing and integration. At a subconscious level their life would be dominated by such questions as "am I safe?" or "is there enough food"? In other words the self has not fully grown beyond that level. Part of the self is left behind in that previous state of traumatised awareness.

There is a further point here. When trauma or difficulty has occurred at a particular stage, traumatic memories can reawaken later in life during periods of stress or transition. For example the infant we just discussed might, as an adult, face a difficult financial situation. He has to take out a large loan to buy a house. At such a time of transition and challenge, earlier unresolved feelings concerning physical safety and welfare will be re-awoken. In the language of psychology, a complex will be activated. The result will be psychological difficulty or physical illness. Of course this period of stress and difficulty also offers an opportunity to address and heal unresolved wounds from the past.

Wounds sustained to body or soul during the course of development can be carried throughout life as underlying tendencies to psychological problems or physical disease. Sometimes these tendencies are dormant, sometimes active.

It is now well known that the earlier in life that conflict or trauma occurs the more fundamental and far reaching will be the effects. We can see then that a holistic therapy, such as homœopathy, is going to have to be able to reach back into the past to bring about healing to such wounds. As far as the developmental model presented here goes, we can say that homœopathy can potentially be of help at *any* of the levels. Successful prescribing will help bring healing to wounded or vulnerable parts of the whole self (as well as to the physical dysfunctions which are the outward expression of such inner problems). In the next chapter we'll come to see just how helpful an understanding of developmental stages can be in understanding patients.

Let's now look at the stages of development in a little more detail. For the sake of cross-discipline continuity I have stayed with the terms that Wilber has used.

Developmental stages

0. Intrauterine existence and birth.

This stage is characterised by symbiosis and dependence. The self of the infant is in a kind of symbiotic union with that of the mother. (Thus the stage is referred to as "0"). In utero the foetus is, as it were, part of the mother. In the early stages of the infant's life the emotional self is also part of the mother's emotional being. The way the mother is with the infant, the way she holds the little one, the way she feels about him or her will lay crucial foundations, not only for the development of the personality, but for the future health or sickness of the individual.

What about birth itself? We know that birth can be traumatic. Indeed in some cases it is life threatening or fatal. Stanislav Grof has shown that individuals carry, deep within the psyche, the memory of the tumultuous and sometimes life threatening experience of birth. Grof has suggested, based on a large body of research and evidence, that the birth experience is *the* formative experience, which shapes much of the individual's future patterns of behaviour and reaction. He reached these conclusions based on his work with thousands of patients. Through regression techniques patients were able to re-enter actual birth experiences, and thence report back the powerful and often life forming experiences they had undergone as they emerged into the world. He has suggested that there are four fundamental phases in the birth process, which he calls basic perinatal matrices.[5] Each stage has its own characteristics and is accompanied by profound physical, emotional and imaginational experiences. Homœopath Harry van der Zee has suggested, based on Grof's work, that a patient's case history, as well as the symptom pictures which arise in the course of homœopathic provings, may be understood as arising from the imprint of the experience of the stages of birth.[6] This is, I believe, an important line of inquiry that deserves to be followed further.

The manner of your birth leaves a deep impression. It informs the way you go about life. The way you are shaped by your birth gives birth to the shape of your life. Being born can bring feelings of loss of continuity, safety and belonging. Birth means that the infant loses the safety and security of the womb, where everything is effortlessly supplied, and is pushed out of this safe haven into a life of uncertainty. Of course much will depend on the love, warmth, nourishment and security, or lack of it, with which parents meet the newcomer to this world.

Thus noting the conditions of birth, along with the mother's state of mind and health during pregnancy and delivery, can be an important consideration in the homœopathic treatment of children, and sometimes of adults as well.

1. Physical/physiocentric self

This is the sensorimotor level of existence. In the first few months of life the infant is identified with the physical world. There is little sense of separation or difference between his or her own physical presence and that of the world. At about four months the infant begins to differentiate between the physical sensations that arise from within its own body, and those that originate from outside. This gives rise to a sense of physical self. This is the first stage in the emergence of consciousness of self. By the age of five to nine months the "hatching" of the physical self should be complete.[7] If this differentiation fails to fully take place the individual may have problems later in life concerned with being able to tell where there own body ends and the environment begins. Pathologies such as autism can be rooted in this developmental stage. Of course difficulties related to this stage of development don't only appear in the form of severe pathologies. Thus in the homœopathic consultation individuals who are in some way stuck at this stage will reveal difficulties connected with their fundamental sense of self, as well as a concern with issues of physical survival and well-being.

2. Emotional/feeling self

In the first year or two of life the infant is identified with the emotional world. There is little sense of difference between self and other on the feeling level. In this sense the infant is almost entirely egocentric. Narcissism rules. The infant is in fusion with its own impulses and the dynamics of the emotional world in which it exists. Wilber writes, "the self is here purely … a libidinal self, a natural-impulsive self. It is one with, in fusion with, the entire vital-emotional dimension of being, both internal and external. It is pushed and pulled by the currents of its vital life, and it does not differentiate itself from the ecological currents of existence." [8]

Between the ages of 15 and 24 months the emotional self begins to differentiate from the emotional environment. A sense of being an emotional self, and thus a separate self begins to emerge. This developmental stage will turn out to be of central importance in our later considerations of the dynamics of health and disease. Psychological birth is now truly underway. At this stage the structure of the emotional self, which will underpin the whole future emotional life of the individual, is being established. Individuals whose suffering is centred at this level will have problems concerned primarily with relationship difficulties. Their emotional boundaries may be damaged, absent or overly protected.

3. Mental/conceptual self

This is the level of the representational mind. It corresponds roughly to what Piaget called the stage of pre-operational cognition.[9] Here we find the capacity to form images, symbols and concepts. It is thought that images emerge at around seven months. Symbols emerge during the second year and are the primary preoccupation of awareness roughly between the ages of two and four years. Concepts are the primary preoccupation between the ages of four and seven years. To give you an idea of the difference between an image, a symbol and a concept, Wilber suggests the following. The image is of just a dog. A symbol, in the sense of the word as used here, denotes our dog, our pet, the one you play with, Bilbo or Pilot or whatever he or she may be called. A concept denotes the understanding that there are many dogs. A concept enables the notion of dogs as a whole.

With the advent of concepts the mental/conceptual self begins to differentiate. We see the emergence of a self with the capacity to hold ideas and concepts of itself and the world.

By the age of seven the foundations of the three fundamental structures of consciousness – physical, emotional, mental – have been laid down.[10]

Wilber again. "The self is now not just a bundle of sensations, and impulses and emotions, it is also a set of symbols and concepts."[11] The self is now living not only in the physical and emotional worlds, but in the world of language and concepts as well.

Problems related to this stage of development will be concerned with the image or concept one has of one self. This does not mean that there will be no physical or emotional dysfunction. It simply means that the focus of the problem, as revealed in the patient's story, will be concerned with issues of identity, self-image, and my notion of the images others have of me. Damage to my self-image will of course carry an emotional charge. Feelings will constellate around this damage. However this is not the same as a wound that is really focused at the feeling level. The latter kind of wound is primarily concerned with issues of relationship, emotional nurture and so on.

Let's take a break now in our review of the developmental stages. As we have reached an important staging post, around the age of seven years old, I'd like to pause and consider a little more the dynamics of repression and splitting. To help us here I'm going to introduce the notion of the shadow.

Shadow

During the development of the self much can get left behind, repressed or denied. Upbringing and education often mean that some form of splitting takes place. The nearer to our unfettered natural being that damage or splitting occurs, in other words the earlier in life, the more far-reaching the consequences are likely to be.

The way you emerge into the world will shape your physical self, your feelings, and your images of self and world. The way the world meets you generates the positive and negative fault lines along which the self-conscious personality develops. This is the way of the world. It is the way that character is formed. It's also the way we're pushed out of shape or wounded.

As the self-conscious "I" is formed, and meets the conditions of the world – family, education, and so on – one can lose the ability to live fully in one-self. Choices are made; avenues get blocked. Parts of one's original whole-ness can become shut down and others relied on too heavily. The influence of family, education and culture can mean contact with roots of vitality, the life of body and soul, can be damaged, compromised or lost.

As the personality develops what happens to the energies that get blocked, the feelings that we repress, the "selves" that can find no place in the world? Unexpressed energies and unfelt feelings can become problematic. Natural drives and feelings need to find their place. If these vital roots become dammed up, then as the personality develops it will be denied the waters and nutrients of the life force. The tree becomes withered. There can be lack of life, lack of creativity, lack of inspiration. On the other hand unaccepted longings and drives must be controlled. This creates rigidity in the personality. Thence change and development must be further resisted. When the wheel of change is resisted, the powers of destruction are never far away.

This is not the same as saying that infantile urges can have free reign. Living in the world means adapting to the conditions of family and society whilst honouring innate life drives at the same time.

What is not accepted, not expressed, not felt, can become buried. This unlived or denied life becomes the poison and sickness of individual and of civilisation, exerting its influence on everyday living from the subconscious. It is a simple truth, confirmed through homœopathic practice, that life has to flow and attain its desire. When denied it becomes a disease-producing poison. This realm of unlived life is what Jung called the shadow – the unexpressed, unfelt and unacknowledged.[12]

Does all this make sense from the perspective of Hahnemann's writings and the basic tenets of homœopathy? Well yes, for Hahnemann equates the vital force with our instinctual nature. In disease the vitality and wisdom of instinct is damaged, denied or lost.

Your life force is the basis of your truth. It is the basis of the knowing of Nature as she is embodied in your constitution. So to lose contact with vital roots is to lose contact with guidance and knowing. Now it may be that the hypnotic effect of the world produced this state of affairs. It is the world that draws us away from inner knowing. However only the individual can claim back inner vitality and knowing. Often this part of ourselves needs to be redeemed from the sleep-inducing state of the world. Disease expresses the way that a person has lost the thread of the knowing of the vital force. Thus healing must involve retracing your steps back to this source of wisdom, which is at the same time the wellspring of your vitality.

Symptoms

The powers of life, when denied or ignored, can become troublesome and disruptive energies, pressing for attention. What isn't accepted thus has to find subconscious channels of expression. What isn't acknowledged or accepted gets in through the back door. What does this mean? It means that these energies appear in the form of unusual sensations and alteration of function. In short they appear as what we homœopaths call symptoms. I'll be devoting a chapter to symptom formation later on. Here I'll simply introduce the subject with a brief look at the form symptoms take.

Feelings

Feelings and emotions that we don't allow ourselves to feel, or that cannot find any expression, get stored up below consciousness. They block the psychic system and can often come out at inappropriate times and in an inappropriate form. Thus one has an outburst about something trivial. The real problem may however be a long stored up resentment. Held back feelings can become toxic to body and soul. This is not the same as saying we should let our feelings rule our lives. However we do need to feel them and honour them.

Dreams

One way that disowned or outlawed elements of your nature try to come into the house of your soul is by appearing in your dreams. It is often said that figures and landscapes in dreams are actually part of the wholeness of your psyche. This is often the case. A dream will often reflect how you really feel about life and which part of yourself is really calling the shots in your behaviour and thoughts.

Body

The body must often give form to forms of being, forms of desire and forms of reaction that somehow cannot find a place within the wholeness of the personality. The body attempts to redress the balance by producing symptoms.

Inner and outer

As we've seen, disease or dysfunction can be observed as alteration of function and behaviour. This is the "outside" of the human holon. Disease can also be imagined (images), felt and sensed from the inside. This is the inner or sub-jective realm of the human holon.

What's important is that the homœopath perceives the inner perceptions of a person and any outer manifestations as a single whole.

However, feelings and sensations are often buried or hidden in a person. They exist beyond the realm of everyday consciousness. People learn to rationalise their feelings and sensations and thus protect themselves from inner pain and uncertainty. If homœopath and patient are to go beyond these rationalisations and enter a space where the patient can *feel* the feelings and *sense* the sensations, then they need to be prepared to journey together beyond the threshold of everyday consciousness. When this happens there is a much better chance that the case will be understood in its entirety (inner and outer), and thus a much better chance of a deep acting similimum being found. I'll be returning to this important aspect of the meeting between homœopath and patient later.

Lets return to the developmental stages.

Developmental stages (continued)

4. The rule/role mind

This is related to what Piaget called the concrete operational stage. In this stage we see the emergence of the capacity to follow rules and take on roles in life. These considerations are the central preoccupation of self-conscious-ness from roughly the ages of six to seven to the ages of eleven to fourteen. Thus this stage takes us, roughly speaking, up to the onset of puberty. Clearly the child has been following rules and taking on roles to a certain extent before the age of six or seven. However at this age the need and ability to do this becomes more central and more pressing. The child becomes less ego-centric and more sociocentric. The child begins to become aware that they belong to a group of other individuals, and that this group is held together by rules. The child more clearly realises that there are other needs and other points of view besides their own. In the education system introduced by Rudolph Steiner, known as Waldorf education, this stage is initiated by the change of teeth, and the child is deemed to be ready for education proper.

In this stage the child develops the capacity for awareness of and care for the immediate group. The child becomes aware of social rules and morals. The child also learns now to follow scripts. This of course strengthens the possibility that the emerging individual will lose touch with or deny their own inner truth. It becomes more possible for the emerging self to participate in collective social or cultural illusions. This is more likely to happen if the individual has been damaged at earlier stages of development. When this stage develops on the basis of a wounded emotional self, the adult individual will be more susceptible to the economic, political and religious illusions perpetrated by powerful groups on the world stage.

Sometimes this stage is referred to as the conventional stage. Before this the child has been "pre-conventional", because not yet really aware of convention. A healthy individual, in as much as health involves being able to feel one's own feelings and think one's own thoughts, must eventually become "post-conventional." [13]

5. Formal-reflexive awareness

Piaget's term for this stage is "formal operational". This is the stage in which the individual develops the capacity to reflect, rather than just accept the rules without question. This stage, roughly coinciding with the onset of puberty, usually begins between the ages of eleven and fifteen. It ushers in the exciting and often difficult period of teenagehood. What's happening?

The emergent individual is for the first time facing and drawing on their own individuality, *in the awareness that they are in fact an individual.* Reflection, and thinking for yourself starts to become possible. The individual can for the first time, as an individual, dream and imagine. Above all the capacity to question and judge begins to emerge (teenagers!), rather than the more or less unconditional acceptance of norms that has preceded this stage. As any parent of teenagers will tell you, the boy or girl of this age can be enormously egocentric, convinced that they are right and that the parents are nothing but ignorant upholders of the status quo. However this is because the individual is, for the first time, really becoming conscious of their own individuality. If this stage is able to unfold in a healthy fashion (remembering that each stage tends to emerge at a certain age, from which time it should go on developing) it gives the individual the ability to know their own thoughts and feelings, as well as the capacity to stand by those thoughts and feelings, even if they are unconventional.

What we see then in this stage is the capacity to reflect on your own truth, honour your own perceptions and dream your own dreams. The individual will of course express their own truth at earlier stages, but in a rather blind and instinctive fashion. Without access to the wellspring of your own imagination, there can be no originality or creativity.

This stage brings the individual to the threshold of adulthood, traditionally set at the age of twenty-one, and now, rightly or wrongly, at eighteen.

6. Vision-logic

This stage represents the emergence of the healthy well-adjusted individual. Well-adjusted in the sense that they are in touch with their own inner being, and well-adjusted in the sense that they can play their part in society. The individual at this stage is capable of being true to themselves as well as serving the good of the whole. For the first time the individual has the capacity for inner authority. Individuals in this stage of development often hold positions of authority in society.

If this stage develops at all, it would, I suggest, first emerge between the ages of twenty-one and forty-two. The development of this stage would then, in health, unfold over the remainder of the person's life.

This stage marks, as it were, the development of a humanitarian self, who may or may not come to embrace the transpersonal levels.

Transpersonal Levels

The vision-logic level is characterised by integration of mind and body and integration in respect to one's place in the world. It paves the way for and merges with the transpersonal.

Transpersonal consciousness ushers in a greater consciousness of the whole. This is the wholeness (spirit, void, unmanifest) that always was and always will be, despite the illusions, trials and sufferings of self-consciousness. It is the undivided, always and only reality. Only relatively few individuals in history have been able to live and have their being at the transpersonal level.

Many of course have breakthrough experiences of the transpersonal. These "peak" experiences can take many forms – realisations of oneness; love for others; a deep experience of presence; complete engagement in a creative pursuit. What do these and other similar experiences have in common? During these moments there is a complete absence of normal self-consciousness. One is taken up in the depth and timelessness of the "now." One is fully present and the everyday sense of self is absent.

Breakthrough into the transpersonal can also come about through suffering. Through trauma or loss the normal self can be pushed beyond its capacity to control and rationalise. There is a breakdown of normal control mechanisms. This breakdown can be pathological or transformative. It can lead to pathological disintegration (which involves collapse to early developmental stages) or to surrender to the reality of the transpersonal Self. This surrender is born on the back of the understanding that all notions of control and choice held by self-consciousness are illusion.

In times of great suffering, as in times of great joy, we may be led to surrender to the will of the transpersonal Self – a will that is beyond the capacity of self-consciousness to know. The realisation that we can only be led, only be guided, is a sign that the transpersonal Self is taking hold of our lives.

Today greater numbers of individuals stand at the threshold of the transpersonal. What are the signs of the awakening to its presence in an individual? There is an awareness of, and an attempt to live with and embrace the opposites within oneself. There is a non-judgemental acceptance of the good and bad, the light and dark, the male and female within oneself. One is attentive to (without judgement) all that arises within and around one. There is more self-knowledge and self-acceptance. One gives oneself over to one's destiny, one's Self.

Wilber, based on the teachings of the Vedantas and other Eastern traditions, suggests four main stages of the transpersonal – the psychic, the subtle, the causal and the non-dual. The psychic level is characterised by the dissolution of the self and a union with nature. At the subtle level of awareness there is union with God (the deity, whichever name it is known by). At the causal level there is realisation of the formless, the creative ground which is the Self of all creation. At the non-dual stage all differentiation between self and other is dissolved. There is only pure unbroken consciousness.

We have now described the journey from stage "0", where there is wholeness, but no self conscious "I", through the stages of emergent self

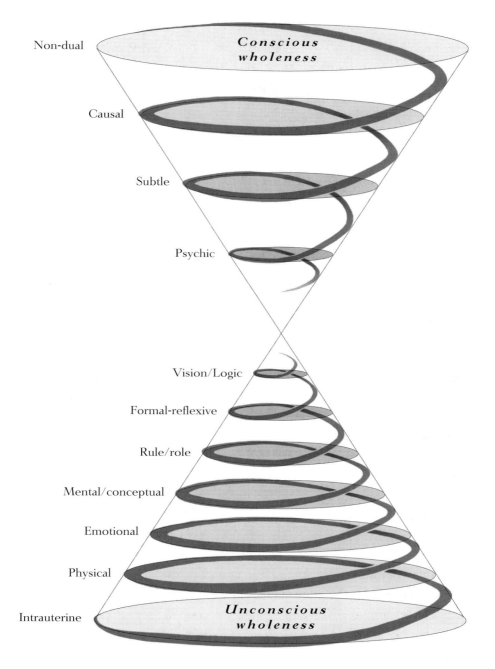

Non-dual

Conscious wholeness

Causal

Subtle

Psychic

Vision/Logic

Formal-reflexive

Rule/role

Mental/conceptual

Emotional

Physical

Intrauterine

Unconscious wholeness

Fig. 3.1 Personal and Transpersonal

As the conscious "I" ascends, the transpersonal Self descends to meet it.

consciousness, to the transpersonal stages of conscious reunion with the once and always wholeness. Originally there was the "I" that didn't know, thence the "I" that knew, and thence knew that it knew. In the end there is the "I" that is not.

Integration

I have spoken of stages of development. However we should not think of these simply as levels one on top of each other. Neither do they replace each other. Rather each stage represents a more embracing form of consciousness that transcends and includes the previous stage. For example the emotional self develops out of and on the basis of the physical self. Without this basis it could not come into being. In health the emotional self doesn't replace the physical self, but transcends and includes it. What actually happens in practice, almost always, is that there is a degree of repression of the consciousness of previous levels. For example as the mental self emerges, with its capacity to conceptualise, feelings may be denied or outlawed. This happens because the needs or the wounds of those previous stages come into conflict with external reality. Repression of difficulties becomes necessary in the face of external demands.

Healthy development asks for integration of previous stages of development. It also asks for increasing integration into the holons of society and culture. An obvious difficulty here is that this outer integration can happen at the expense of inner integration. In other words the fulfilment of outer obligation can lead to denial of self. In this scenario the self – the emotional self for example – remains wounded and unable to develop. When this happens the adult individual, while supposedly an adult as far as the external world goes, remains a child. Healthy development asks that one's development as part of a larger whole goes hand in hand with healthy inner development.

Other models

It is important to remember that this is only a model, an aid to the perception of reality and not the reality itself. Reality itself is always far more inventive, flexible and creative, than even the most sophisticated models could ever be.

There are other models. Freud spoke of the oral, anal and sexual stages of infant and child development. He also emphasised the conflict between the id – the presence of the instinctual drives within the individual – and the superego. The superego represents the presence of society's rules within the individual's psyche. The conflict between these two generates the battleground of the ego and gives rise to neurosis.

Abraham Maslow's famous model of the hierarchy of human needs has much in common with what has been discussed so far. It is also striking that Hahnemann, in his directions on the gathering of case data, also recognised the broad outlines of the developmental model used in this chapter.

Wilber	Hahnemann	Maslow
Vision logic		Self actualization
	Sexual function?	
Formal reflexive		Aesthetic needs
	Civic and	
Rule/role	domestic relationships	
		Cognitive needs
Mental/conceptual	Mental and	Esteem needs
	emotional character	
Emotional/feeling		Love and belonging
Physical	Body constitution	Safety needs
Intrauterine/birth	Sexual function?	Physiological needs

Fig. 3.2 Comparison of Wilber, Hahnemann and Maslow[14]

The model of the development of self consciousness used here is a seven level map. This will be an important consideration when we come onto homœopathic theory. Our map also recognises the importance of a seven-year cycle (concepts, age 4-7; reflective/creative, age 11-15 etc.).

In the seven year rhythm – 7, 14, 21, 28, 35, 42, 49, 56, 63, 70, 77, 84 – we can recognise many crucial stages such as puberty, mid-life and so on. Astrologers also recognise important developmental cycles associated with the movement of the outer planets, which often synchronise with the seven-year cycle. For example Saturn returns to the natal position at around the age of 27 to 28.

The model presented in this chapter tallies well with the homœopathic theory that we'll come to in the next chapter. It also includes the transpersonal. In other words it represents stages of personal development as well as transpersonal development. Conventional psychological research has tended to focus on the stages of personal development. Spiritual traditions, on the other hand, tend to focus on spiritual development. This model attempts to embrace both realities.

In the next chapter we'll get more specifically homœopathic.

Chapter 4:
Homœopathic Correspondences

In the last chapter I introduced a developmental model in an attempt to further our understanding of the dynamics of health and sickness in the human individual. I'd like now to take these ideas a step further. If the developmental process is something essential in the human being, and if disturbances in the developmental process are essential to human sickness, then we would expect to find evidence of this in the homœopathic theoretical framework. Let's see if this might be so.

The ideas presented in this and the next chapter build on the pioneering work of two modern homœopathic physician philosophers, Rajan Sankaran and Jan Scholten.

Periodic Table

Scholten sees the periodic table as a single dynamic pattern.[1] Understanding the place of each element within the overall pattern allows us to gain a fuller understanding of remedies prepared from the different elements and compounds.

Let's just summarise his ideas. According to him each period (horizontal row) has a certain theme. He names each period according to the major remedy in that period. For example the themes of the fourth period (the Ferrum series) are described by such words as task, work, duty, trade, skill, practical, order, rules, control, criticised, failure, fault, guilt, police. We can see that this series relates to the rule/role stage of development.

Group

Group	1 / 1A	2 / 2A	3 / 3B	4 / 4B	5 / 5B	6 / 6B	7 / 7B	8 / 8B	9 / 8B	10 / –	11 / 1B	12 / 2B	13 / 3A	14 / 4A	15 / 5A	16 / 6A	17 / 7A	18 / 8A
1	1 **H** Hydrogen (1)																	2 **He** Helium (2)
2	3 **Li** Lithium (2,1)	4 **Be** Beryllium (2,2)											5 **B** Boron (2,3)	6 **C** Carbon (2,4)	7 **N** Nitrogen (2,5)	8 **O** Oxygen (2,6)	9 **F** Fluorine (2,7)	10 **Ne** Neon (2,8)
3	11 **Na** Sodium (2,8,1)	12 **Mg** Magnesium (2,8,2)											13 **Al** Aluminum (2,8,3)	14 **Si** Silicon (2,8,4)	15 **P** Phosphorus (2,8,5)	16 **S** Sulfur (2,8,6)	17 **Cl** Chlorine (2,8,7)	18 **Ar** Argon (2,8,8)
4	19 **K** Potassium (2,8,8,1)	20 **Ca** Calcium (2,8,8,2)	21 **Sc** Scandium (2,8,9,2)	22 **Ti** Titanium (2,8,10,2)	23 **V** Vanadium (2,8,11,2)	24 **Cr** Chromium (2,8,13,1)	25 **Mn** Manganese (2,8,13,2)	26 **Fe** Iron (2,8,14,2)	27 **Co** Cobalt (2,8,15,2)	28 **Ni** Nickel (2,8,16,2)	29 **Cu** Copper (2,8,18,1)	30 **Zn** Zinc (2,8,18,2)	31 **Ga** Gallium (2,8,18,3)	32 **Ge** Germanium (2,8,18,4)	33 **As** Arsenic (2,8,18,5)	34 **Se** Selenium (2,8,18,6)	35 **Br** Bromine (2,8,18,7)	36 **Kr** Krypton (2,8,18,8)
5	37 **Rb** Rubidium (2,8,18,8,1)	38 **Sr** Strontium (2,8,18,8,2)	39 **Y** Yttrium (2,8,18,9,2)	40 **Zr** Zirconium (2,8,18,10,2)	41 **Nb** Niobium (2,8,18,12,1)	42 **Mo** Molybdenum (2,8,18,13,1)	43 **Tc** Technetium (2,8,18,13,2)	44 **Ru** Ruthenium (2,8,18,15,1)	45 **Rh** Rhodium (2,8,18,16,1)	46 **Pd** Palladium (2,8,18,18,0)	47 **Ag** Silver (2,8,18,18,1)	48 **Cd** Cadmium (2,8,18,18,2)	49 **In** Indium (2,8,18,18,3)	50 **Sn** Tin (2,8,18,18,3)	51 **Sb** Antimony (2,8,18,18,4)	52 **Te** Tellurium (2,8,18,18,5)	53 **I** Iodine (2,8,18,18,6)	54 **Xe** Xenon (2,8,18,18,8)
6	55 **Cs** Cesium (2,8,18,18,8,1)	56 **Ba** Barium (2,8,18,18,8,2)	57 to 71	72 **Hf** Hafnium (2,8,18,32,10,2)	73 **Ta** Tantalum (2,8,18,32,11,2)	74 **W** Tungsten (2,8,18,32,12,2)	75 **Re** Rhenium (2,8,18,32,13,2)	76 **Os** Osmium (2,8,18,32,14,2)	77 **Ir** Iridium (2,8,18,32,15,2)	78 **Pt** Platinum (2,8,18,32,16,2)	79 **Au** Gold (2,8,18,32,18,1)	80 **Hg** Mercury (2,8,18,32,18,1)	81 **Tl** Thallium (2,8,18,32,18,2)	82 **Pb** Lead (2,8,18,32,18,3)	83 **Bi** Bismuth (2,8,18,32,18,4)	84 **Po** Polonium (2,8,18,32,18,5)	85 **At** Astatine (2,8,18,32,18,7)	86 **Rn** Radon (2,8,18,32,18,8)
7	87 **Fr** Francium (2,8,18,32,18,8,1)	88 **Ra** Radium (2,8,18,32,18,8,1)	89 to 103	104 **Rf** Rutherfordium	105 **Db** Dubnium (2,8,18,32,32,10,2)	106 **Sg** Seaborgium (2,8,18,32,32,12,2)	107 **Bh** Bohrium (2,8,18,32,32,12,2)	108 **Hs** Hassium (2,8,18,32,32,13,2)	109 **Mt** Meitnerium (2,8,18,32,32,13,2)	110 **Uun** Ununilium (2,8,18,32,32,16,2)	111 **Uuu** Unununium (2,8,18,32,32,17,1)	112 **Uub** Ununbium (2,8,18,32,32,18,2)	113	114 **Uuq** Ununquadium	115	116 **Uuh** Ununhexium	117	118 **Uuo** Ununoctium

Lanthanum:

57 **La** Lanthanum (2,8,18,18,9,2)	58 **Ce** Cerium (2,8,18,19,9,2)	59 **Pr** Praseodymium (2,8,18,21,8,2)	60 **Nd** Neodymium (2,8,18,22,8,2)	61 **Pm** Promethium (2,8,18,23,8,2)	62 **Sm** Samarium (2,8,18,24,8,2)	63 **Eu** Europium (2,8,18,25,8,2)	64 **Gd** Gadolinium (2,8,18,25,9,2)	65 **Tb** Terbium (2,8,18,27,8,2)	66 **Dy** Dysprosium (2,8,18,28,8,2)	67 **Ho** Holmium (2,8,18,29,8,2)	68 **Er** Erbium (2,8,18,29,8,2)	69 **Tm** Thulium (2,8,18,30,8,2)	70 **Yb** Ytterbium (2,8,18,31,8,2)	71 **Lu** Lutetium (2,8,18,32,9,2)

Actinium:

89 **Ac** Actinium (2,8,18,32,18,9,2)	90 **Th** Thorium (2,8,18,32,18,10,2)	91 **Pa** Protactinium (2,8,18,32,20,9,2)	92 **U** Uranium (2,8,18,32,21,9,2)	93 **Np** Neptunium (2,8,18,32,21,9,2)	94 **Pu** Plutonium (2,8,18,32,23,8,2)	95 **Am** Americium (2,8,18,32,24,8,2)	96 **Cm** Curium (2,8,18,32,25,9,2)	97 **Bk** Berkelium (2,8,18,32,25,8,2)	98 **Cf** Californium (2,8,18,32,26,8,2)	99 **Es** Einsteinium (2,8,18,32,28,8,2)	100 **Fm** Fermium (2,8,18,32,29,8,2)	101 **Md** Mendelevium (2,8,18,32,30,8,2)	102 **No** Nobelium (2,8,18,32,31,8,2)	103 **Lr** Lawrencium (2,8,18,32,32,9,2)

Fig. 4.1 Periodic table

There are seven horizontal rows called periods. Scholten calls these series. The eighteen vertical columns are called groups. Scholten calls them stages. Groups 1-18 were previously known by other notations, 1a, 2a, 3b etc.

The number shown with each element is the atomic number and refers to the number of positively charged protons (as well as neutrons) in the nucleus and negatively charged electrons orbiting the nucleus. For example hydrogen has one proton and one electron. Helium has two of each.

The Lanthanide series and Actinide series are shown as a separate block at the bottom of the chart. The Lanthanides fall between 57 and 72, and the Actinides between 89 and 104. They are shown like this to make the chart more compact; also because they are chemically similar to each other.

The middle block of the chart are known as the transition elements. Again they are similar structurally and chemically. For example cobalt is similar to both iron and nickel. Each is strongly magnetic, and their melting points are similar. Thus they are also similar homœopathically.

Elements 110 to 118 are suspected but either undiscovered or unverified.

Scholten has made some significant changes to the conventional layout of the chart. Boron is moved from group 15 to 3;

carbon from 14 to 10; aluminium from 13 to 3; silicon from 14 to 10. Based on their homœopathic characteristics, he feels that this is where they should be placed.

The electrons are arranged in shells around the nucleus. All the elements in the first period have one shell, all the elements in the second period have two shells, all those in the third period have three shells and so on. Thus as you go down the chart the elements get heavier. For example hydrogen (period one) is a light gas, and lead (period six) is a heavy metal. The elements of period seven are so heavy that the nucleus is disintegrating. They are radioactive.

Throughout the chart the differences and similarities in the properties of the elements are reflected in the homœopathic pictures. Aurum is a much "heavier" picture than Natrum muriaticum.

Generally speaking the number of electrons in the outer shells of the elements increases as you move from left to right. Thus sodium has one electron in its outer (third) shell, magnesium has two, aluminium three, silicon four and so on.

Elements in the same vertical column have similar properties. For example sodium and potassium are highly reactive. Copper, silver and gold are excellent conductors of heat and electricity. The halogens (group 17) are similar both chemically and homœopathically.

Elements next to each other horizontally can also be similar. For example iridium and platinum are similar and are found together in nature. They are both used in jewellery and in precision instruments. They are both noble metals, resistant to oxidation and corrosion.

The chemical reactivity of an element is related to its atomic number, and particularly to the number of electrons in the outer shell. To be stable an element need eight electrons in its outer shell. To achieve this elements combine and share electrons. Just like people elements are attracted together to form stable combinations. For example sodium has one electron in its outer shell and so needs to combine with an element which needs to make up it's eight. This makes sodium reactive and looking to combine. Sodium people suffer from disappointment in relationship. Sodium needs to find someone to join in with. Chlorine on the other hand has seven electrons in its outer shell. It needs to gain one. Thus when sodium and chlorine get married they combine their one and seven to make eight – a stable whole. The result is sodium chloride – common salt. Chlorine needs to keep this one extra electron. Chlorine people are sensitive to let down and betrayal.

One last point. Think of the atom not as an object, but as a pattern of dynamic movement, with protons and electrons as vortices (particle) or ripples (waves) of motion in the underlying quantum field.

Furthermore each series is divided into stages (a maximum of eighteen, being the maximum number of elements, discounting for now the additional elements normally shown as a separate block at the bottom of the periodic table, found in one horizontal row). These stages represent the different stages of the unfolding of the theme of the period. This sequence, which he sees as a wave pattern, represents the beginning, the establishment and the decline of the theme of that period. So, according to our developmental model, the fourth period would represent the beginning, the establishment and the decline of the rule/role mind.

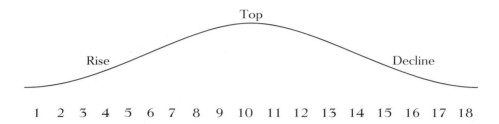

Fig. 4.2 Periodic wave pattern (after Scholten, 1996, p. 29)

What is of particular note from our point of view is that Scholten himself has suggested a developmental sequence. In the chart given below, as well as giving a theme for each period he gives a corresponding age and area of awareness (body, house, village, etc.).

Series	Theme	Age	Area	Sense	Tissue
Hydrogen	Being	Foetus	Spaceless	Smell?	
Carbon	I	Child	Body	Touch?	Skin
Silicium	Other	Teenager	House		Connective tissue
Ferrum	Work	Adult	Village		Muscle, Blood
Silver	Ideas	Middle age	Town	Speech	Nerves
Gold	Leadership	Ripe	Country	Vision	Bone
Uranium	Magus	Old age	Universe	Intuition	Bone marrow

Fig. 4.3 The seven series (from Scholten, 1996, p. 21)

The age column suggests a developmental sequence. At a glance we can see that the themes resemble the key ideas related to each stage of the development of consciousness discussed in the last chapter. The area column also suggests a developmental sequence in the sense that it suggests the sphere with which each subsequent stage of developing self-consciousness becomes identified with. In this sense each period (moving down the table) represents a further expansion of consciousness (body, house, village, etc.). He then goes on to suggest that the periodic table, when viewed as a spiral, can be seen as a model of the *expansion of human consciousness.*

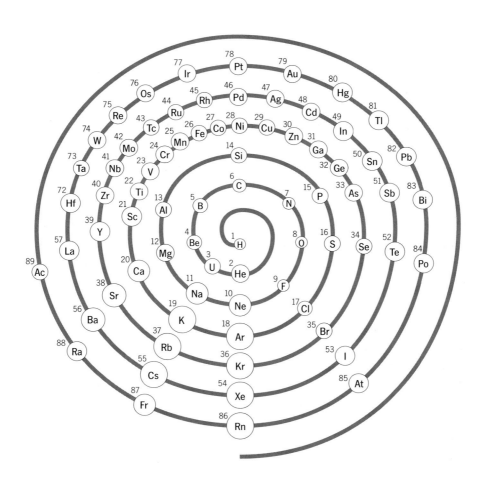

Fig. 4.4 The periodic spiral (after Scholten, 1996, p. 19)

The ideas put forward here build on Jan Scholten's work. We have seen so far that the development and differentiation of human self-consciousness is a fundamental necessity on the path to deeper and broader awareness and the fulfilment of human destiny. However there is also a disruptive tendency within the developmental process that dismembers primal being and knowing. Healing must not only address this damage but must also help us to become conscious participants in the wholeness of ourselves and the world. Here and in the next chapter we will see how the stages of development with their accompanying wounds and dysfunctions are reflected in the periods and remedies of the periodic table.

I don't propose to go through every remedy, nor do I propose to give an exhaustive picture of each remedy. Rather the purpose here is to take a number of key remedies (either as elements or salts) and simply give an outline of the essential themes of the remedy. As we do this we'll relate those themes to the sequence of the development and differentiation of consciousness.

0. Intrauterine/birth stage

This is a stage of incarnation, conception and symbiotic unity with the mother, and the beginnings of the emergence of self-consciousness. This stage corresponds with the first period of the periodic table. Among the key ideas given by Scholten for the Hydrogen series are: being; to be or not to be; incarnation; outside space/time and incarnation into space/time. We can think of the first period then as corresponding to the pre-birth stage (outside space and time), conception and intrauterine existence, through to birth.

Hydrogen

In the proving of Hydrogen conducted by Jeremy Sherr, feelings of unreality, of not being in the world, of not being in the body were reported.[2] There were feelings of universal love. Time seemed like an aeon. There were also feelings of being pulled down (conception?). Thus we can say that hydrogen, the first element of the first period, represents the transition from timelessness to time, from formlessness to form, and from spirit to matter. There were delusions of pregnancy, which we could take as a symbolic expression of the first emergence of the self-conscious "I".

We have seen that as consciousness begins to differentiate, the infant moves from a condition of complete symbiosis with the mother (universal love) to the dawning sense of a separate self, and thus also a sense of other. We find in Hydrogen symptoms of being separate, not belonging and isolation. These feelings ultimately give rise to feelings of despair, hopelessness and suicide.

There were also symptoms of confusion between left and right, and confusion of sexual identity. These symptoms seem to symbolise the stage of development in which consciousness is only just beginning to differentiate. When you incarnate you leave behind wholeness and take on a male or female identity. You are also equipped with a brain with two cerebral hemispheres, the left being more concerned with discrimination and the right more with wholeness. Thus confusion between left and right arises out of the conflict between symbiotic wholeness and the need for a differentiated self-consciousness.

In summary then the Hydrogen picture represents birth into the world of duality. One could say that this also involves the soul's decision (need?) to incarnate or not. The symptoms constellate around incarnation and conception, intrauterine existence, symbiotic unity and birth.

1. Physical stage

This stage of development sees the emergence of the physical sense of self. It corresponds with the second period of the periodic table. Among the key ideas given by Scholten for the carbon series are: the first emergence of a sense of "I"; body, life and instinct; material existence.

This series represents the first and fundamental differentiation of consciousness, the first awareness of difference, of I and other. It is the first and most basic (body) level of discriminating consciousness. Thus one's most basic judgements concerning self and other, good and bad and so on are formed at this level.

Borax (Sodium biborate)

This salt, a combination of sodium and boron, is interesting from our point of view. Boron is the third element along of the second period. Boron is normally placed in column 13 of the periodic table, formerly designated as column 3a.

Scholten suggests that it can legitimately be placed in column 3 immediately adjacent to Beryllium. The remedy Borax is famous for fear or anxiety from downward motion. In our schema this would correspond with the process of birth and entry into the external physical world. The remedy also contains the sodium element. Sodium is concerned with feelings of loss. Thus the theme of Borax might be sense of loss (sodium) through birth (downward motion). Borax has the symptom: fear of falling in children; must hold on to mother or nurse.

Carbon

Carbon has atomic number 6. It is normally placed in column 14, formerly known as 4a. Scholten suggests that it belongs in column 10 with silicon, nickel, palladium and platinum. The remedy Graphites is an almost pure form of carbon. In the remedy we find symptoms concerned with the physical basis of human life, with the meeting of basic survival needs:

- anxiety; eating; amel.
- avarice
- delusions, imaginations; unfortunate, he is
- fear; general; poverty

What can we make of this? Let's turn here to carbon and the life of plants. Through photosynthesis plants convert atmospheric carbon dioxide into complex carbon compounds known as carbohydrates. Sugars, starches and cellulose are carbohydrates. Plant tissue is made up of carbohydrates. Plants get their energy from sunlight and from the chemical breakdown of sugars. Animals eat plants or other animals and obtain their carbon in that way. We burn fossil (carbon) fuels for energy and warmth. In other words the breakdown of carbon compounds releases energy. This is the energy required to drive the metabolic processes of organic life. Carbohydrates are the basis of the food chain. Carbon compounds constitute the fuel that is burnt on the fires of life. They make up the fuel for the vitality of life. Thus a basic concern of Graphites, and in various different ways the carbon salts, might be, "Is there enough fuel?"or "Will I survive?"

Concerning the carbon remedies in general, Sankaran writes, "the basic theme of carbon… is the… fear of death with the need for a vital reaction (activity) in order to survive."[3] This basic issue will be modified according to the salt in question (Calcarea carbonica, Natrum carbonicum etc.).

In the everyday human world survival means food, fuel for the fire, money, and so on. No food, you starve. No fuel, you get cold, and perhaps die. To get fuel one must work. If you don't work to earn money to put fuel on your fire and food in your belly, you die (before the advent of the welfare state anyway).

In the mythological imagination the intrauterine stage is symbolised by the Garden of Eden. There is blissful symbiosis until the eating of the apple brings awareness of sexual difference (Hydrogen). Adam and Eve have to leave the garden (birth) and survive "in the sweat of thy face" by tilling the soil (Genesis, chapter 3, verse 19). This threshold corresponds to the carbon phase of the carbon series.

There is a general point I should make here about provings and the symptom pictures displayed by patients. I am suggesting that proving pictures, and disease pictures displayed by patients, do in fact constellate around problematic developmental stages. However, the symptoms that emerge often don't directly relate to the developmental stage in question because the feelings and perceptions of that stage are long since buried in the unconscious psyche. There they lie as dormant impressions and anxieties that nevertheless have a gravitational pull on the everyday consciousness of the individual. When these unconscious complexes are activated in an everyday situation or in a proving, then the individual experiences that complex, not in its original form, but in a form that makes sense in the (adult) individual's current life. Thus the underlying anxiety about physical existence found in Graphites, translates in the language of the patient's or prover's current consciousness, into "fear of poverty." What in the infant was a dim sense of "am I going to make it or not?" becomes in the adult, "I must keep working, or face the consequences which are poverty and death."

Graphites is also known for its indecision and anxiety over the slightest thing:

- Mind; anxiety; trifles, about
- Mind; irresolution, indecision; trifles, about

Scholten has suggested that these individuals are uncertain over values. The carbon series corresponds to the differentiation of physical consciousness, a bodily sense of self. Once this differentiation starts, once awareness of separation dawns, the way is open for primal value judgements as to what is good or bad (the "good" being what is good for survival, and the "bad" being what is bad for survival). It is as though the Graphites individual cannot make the simplest of judgements (decisions) without awakening the primal survival anxiety characteristic of this stage.

Fluorine
Staying with the second period (of the periodic table) and the physical developmental stage, what can we make of the remedy Fluoric Acid, which owes its picture partly to fluorine and partly to the presence of hydrogen? Fluorine lies in column 17, near the end of the Carbon series. Thus we would expect the remedy to be concerned with the end phase of the physical stage of development. Lets look at some of the listed mind symptoms first:

- adulterous
- aversion; family members, to
- aversion; friends, to
- aversion; parents, to
- aversion; wife, to his
- aversion; women, to
- delusions, imaginations; betrothal, engagement must be broken
- delusions, imaginations; children, thinks he must drive, out of the house
- delusions, imaginations; marriage, must dissolve
- indifference, apathy; business affairs, to
- indifference, apathy; loved ones, to
- indifference, apathy; relations, to
- lasciviousness, lustfulness; ogling women on the street

In Phatak we find, "Aversion; to his own family, to those loved best; becomes interested and converses pleasantly with strangers. Inability to realize responsibility."[4]

This is the stage where consciousness should progress from being centred in the body to being centred in the feelings. It is necessary to transcend the purely material. If there is a problem at this stage the individual remains, as it were, materialistically self-centred. They need to progress to relationship with another. They need to, but can't. Hence the preoccupation with sex without commitment, without responsibility.

The eminent American homœopath Elizabeth Wright Hubbard put it like this:

"Fickle Fluoric acid. Casanova. A charming, fickle butterfly, the man about town who ogles women in the street, the one-night-stand young man with a yen for variety and a great love of strangers. It is a male remedy, or one for mannish women, for the debauchee, trying to prove his manhood through lecherousness and variety." [5]

Among the key words given by Scholten for fluorine are: money, glamour, smooth, shiny, hard (like the enamel of the teeth), possessions, sex. [6] It has been observed that the Fluoric acid individual tends to be materialistic and have difficulty with emotional bonds. [7] They are concerned with the physicality of money and sex.

It is as though body consciousness is no longer confined to its boundaries. "Increased ability to exercise his muscles, without fatigue, regardless of most excessive heat of summer or cold of winter." [8] This transcending of the boundaries of physical consciousness should lead into the more inclusive awareness of the emotional self.

Emotional self

We move now to the next stage of development, the differentiation of the emotional self. The primary issue here is no longer physical survival, but the awareness of self and other in relationship. The key issues here are bonding, nurture and the making and breaking of love relationships. The third stage of development (numbered two in last chapter's map) coincides with the beginning of the third period of the periodic table. So let's start with the Natrums.

Sodium

Sodium is found mainly in the blood and the extra cellular fluids. Sodium effects fluid balance in the body. Imbalance of sodium levels lead to fluid imbalances such as changes in blood volume, oedema, thirst and increased urine. The tissue fluids, where sodium is mainly found, provide the external environment of the cells of the body.

All life on this planet has its origins in the ocean. Early life internalised the oceanic medium. Thus the tissue fluids, along with lymph and blood plasma, can be said to be the internalised ocean. The tissue fluid is the matrix in which the individual cells live.

Sodium, then, is concerned with water and flow. The Natrum homœo-pathic pictures reveal that sodium is also related to the psychological counterpart of water, namely feelings and feeling relationships (see Chapter 9). Sankaran writes, "In the Natrum side we see this marked desire to form and maintain a relationship especially on a one to one level." [9] The issue becomes bonding and separation at a feeling level. As the emotional self differentiates, the issue is no longer simply physical presence or physical survival. There is a dawning awareness of other as well as of self. This brings with it the longing for union, bonding, care, nurture. Thus we have the well-known Natrum symptoms of loss, sadness, grief and disappointed love.

It is interesting to note that the Natrum salts produce many symptoms around the mouth such as various kinds of eruptions and numbness. There are also ailments after coition. The mouth is the place of the primary bond with the mother. It is through the mouth that the child receives the mother's nourishment as well as a sense of emotional nurture and connection. The sexual embrace awakens feelings of love and connection, but can also bring feelings of isolation and loss, for every embrace must lead to a parting.

The Natrum salts represent the first phase in the emergence of the emotional self.

Magnesium

As the differentiation of the emotional self proceeds what would we now expect? If the infant is loved and cared for by a "good enough" mother, then the next stage of the emergence of self-consciousness should not be particularly problematic or traumatic. However it can also be the case that as the awareness of separateness grows greater, so does the anxiety. This brings us to the Magnesium salts.

Sankaran writes, "The Magnesium feeling is that the person doesn't get the care, protection and nourishment that he needs. It is the state of an infant dependent on the mother for nourishment, care, security, and support, but who has been abandoned by his parents." [10] The rubric is:

- forsaken feeling; beloved by his parents, wife, friends, feels is not being

As the self separates further from the mother, both physically and emotionally, the susceptibility to rejection can become greater.

Temper tantrums begin to appear typically in the second year of life, often with the breaking through of the teeth. Chamomilla is often indicated here. Magnesia carbonica is recorded as being complementary to Chamomilla. Repeated Chamomilla episodes point to Magnesia carbonica as a possible constitutional remedy. The Magnesiums themselves are remedies for slow dentition.

Anyone who has witnessed the rage and frustration of the Chamomilla child will get a sense of what's involved here. The teeth introduce the potential for power and aggression – aggression in the infant against the world, particularly the mother, who by now may well be turning out to be a "bad mother" as well as a "good mother", because, as well as giving warmth, nourishment and so on, she seems to desert or threaten the infant. We can imagine that the emerging self is torn by the conflict between aggression on the one hand, and, on the other, the need to appease the mother on whom he is so dependent. Magnesia carbonica is described (resembling Chamomilla) as violent, ill-tempered, erratic, fearful and depressed.[11] There can also be tremendous anxiety.[12] Vithoulkas notes that the Magnesia carbonica individual is a peacemaker who is upset by quarrelling.[13]

Being a Carbonicum (fuel, physical survival, etc.), there are issues in Magnesia carbonica concerning food and nourishment. In particular there is aggravation from milk, including mother's milk. Mother's milk is the nourishment on which one is so dependent, even though that primal bond must be given up. Kent found that orphans in an orphanage were wasting away until they received this remedy.[14]

Magnesium represents a further phase in the development of the emotional self. The emphasis is now more on the conflict between dependence and independence.

The mental/conceptual self

Beyond Magnesium we leave behind the birth of the emotional self. The next stage is the emergence of the mental/conceptual self with its capacity to retain images and concepts, as well as use language. This brings us to the structure of consciousness that is going to emerge and establish itself between approximately the second and sixth year. We should find that the remedies we now encounter in the periodic table are no longer first and foremost concerned with emotional well-being. Rather they are concerned with the image one has of oneself, and the images others have of you. Thus the next group of remedies are concerned with identity, self-image and status.

The psychological "I"

There is a point that needs to be clarified here before we move on. Up to now each stage of development (including its phases of emergence, establishment and decline) has corresponded to a period of the periodic table (Hydrogen series equals conception/intrauterine existence/birth; Carbon series equals birth and differentiation of the physical self).

The physical stage is followed by the next two stages, the emotional and the mental/conceptual. The emotional stage corresponds to the beginning of the third series (Natrum, Magnesium), and the mental/conceptual stage corresponds to the middle and end of the third series (Alumina, Silica, Phosphorus, Sulphur etc.).

O.K., so we've got two stages of development corresponding to one series, whereas previous and subsequent stages more or less each correspond to a period of the periodic table. What can we make of this?

Among the key ideas given by Scholten for the Silica series (third series) are: relationships with another, with family, with siblings, with partner; love and rejection; relationship and communication; language, learning, talking, reading, writing; presentation and appearance.[15]

If we look at this carefully, something becomes clear. These key ideas show a sequential development from the stage of feelings and emotions, where relationships are the key issue, to the mental/conceptual stage where language, communication, learning, presentation and self-image are important. When it comes to the third period, then, we are dealing with two stages of development, the emotional and the mental/conceptual. Can we clarify this further?

It is out of our feeling relationships that we begin to form concepts of ourselves and the world. Thus the emotional and mental stages taken together form the birth, development and decline of the psychological "I". The emphasis on the birth, establishment and decline of the psychological self corresponds to the third series of the periodic table.

Of course, the psychological self does not decline as such. What is meant here is that in the healthy course of development the exclusive identification with the psychological self (emotional/mental) should give way to identification with the wider scope and possibilities of the next developmental stage, the rule/role mind, in which the self becomes aware of the presence of the group. Problems arise in any stage when the self becomes identified with that stage (for example being a self around which everything revolves) and, because of clinging to this identification, is unable to move on to the wider and deeper possibilities of subsequent stages of development.

The next element in our survey, aluminium, can be said to stand at the end of the emotional stage and the beginning of the mental/conceptual stage. Thus the remedy Alumina has, so to speak, symptoms of ending and beginning.

Alumina
This remedy is aluminium oxide. It owes its symptoms to the presence of oxygen as well as aluminium. Aluminium is normally placed in group 13 of the periodic table, formerly known as group 3a. Scholten places it in group 3, next to magnesium and below boron. Let's list some of the well-known mind symptoms:

- blood or a knife, cannot look at
- confusion of mind; identity, as to his; own, as if it were not his
- courageous
- defiant
- delusions, imaginations; consciousness, belongs to another
- delusions, imaginations; says something, somebody else has said it, when he

- delusions, imaginations; body, body parts; head; belongs to another
- fear; general; blood, of
- fear; general; impulses, of his own
- fear; general; knives, of
- fear; general; self-control, losing
- impulsive
- injure; herself, himself, feels could
- kill, desire to; knife; sight of a, at; gun, or a
- kill, desire to; sudden impulse to
- suicidal disposition; knife, with

We can immediately see a number of themes. Identity; control and loss of control (impulsive); violence (violent impulses, suicidal).

Let's turn to Sankaran again. He paints a picture of suppression of identity. "The patient doesn't even know to whom his head belongs. He feels as if somebody else thinks for him, and he can't think for himself." [16] Clearly we're in the mental/conceptual realm here. Sankaran points out that parental control is strong and the child can become impulsive or violent. He continues, "Control is a big theme in Alumina. A lot of problems have to do with control – control of the body, of the limbs, impulses, a fear of losing control. As the mental will has been undermined (symptom: weak will), so also the will is taken away from the muscles too, and he can't move properly…He feels he needs to be hard and rigid in order to keep up his identity."

What can we make of all this as a developmental situation? As the mental/ conceptual self differentiates, we see self-identity becoming the central issue. Let's try to put ourselves in the shoes of the child around the age of four or five. There is no longer simply a physical or feeling sense of self, but a dawning *concept or image* of self. I am I…but I am still small and my parents are big and powerful. I know myself to be myself, but I must also conform to the ideas imposed by my more powerful parents. (Mental/conceptual identity at this stage is still only embryonic.) The unconscious thought process might run like this. Can I be myself, have my own thoughts, know my own mind, or must I conform to what others expect of me? If I am to know my own mind I must fight against this authority that is trying to think for me, thus I must be "courageous", "defiant" and "rigid." At the same time because I am still dependent I must conform to parental ways of thinking. This means I must control myself. I must particularly control the violence I feel towards my controlling parents who don't allow me to be myself. I must control murderous impulses.

However the mental/conceptual self is in its early stages, and self-control has yet to be really established. Thus the unschooled impulses of the vital/emotional self still break through with ease.

What happens to violent impulses that must be repressed? They get turned inward towards oneself:

- injure; herself, himself, feels could
- suicidal disposition; knife, with

Thus we might say that Alumina is the bridge from the emotional self to the mental/conceptual self. Identity is not yet established and the impulses of the emotional self must be controlled. Let's turn to Silica.

Silica
Silicon lies next to aluminium. It is normally placed in group 14, formerly known as group 4a. Scholten has moved it, along with carbon, to group 10. Homœopathic Silica is, like Alumina, an oxide. Alumina has fear of knives, Silica fear of pins and pointed things.

One of the forms of Silica is flint. When man the toolmaker appeared on the evolutionary scene some two million years ago, he began to fashion remarkable tools for cutting and scraping by chipping away at flint. These first cutting instruments would eventually become, after several hundred thousand years, beautifully tooled arrow and spearheads. Man the toolmaker was really man the cutter. The arrival of the ability to cut was an expression of an increased ability to manipulate the world, which, as it happens, appears along with a significantly larger brain.[17]

With Silica we are well and truly into the rational world, the world of analysis. It is through analysis that we, as it were, cut up the world. We divide it up in order to understand it and control it. This we might say is the world of Silica. We know that the Silica individual can be hung up on overly detailed analysis:

- conscientious about trifles

There is too much attention to detail.

In the Silica phase the conceptual mind is really establishing itself. Silica is an intellectual: [18]

- ailments from; work; mental; writing; reading, and
- theorising

Here we have moved on from the identity crisis of Alumina. Now there is a need to feel that you are doing things correctly, and that you are being seen to do things correctly. Let's look at some of the relevant symptoms:

- ailments from; anticipation, foreboding, presentiment; stage-fright
- ailments from; egotism
- anticipation; general; examination, before
- confidence; want of self
- confusion of mind; identity, as to his
- fear; general; failure, of
- fear; general; undertaking anything
- timidity; public, about appearing in; talk, to

What are we dealing with here? Let's summarise. Ego identity in the sense of being a mental/conceptual self; self esteem and the esteem of others; issues of confidence in oneself; having one's own thoughts and ideas, but unsure if they are correct, thus internal conflict:

- antagonism; herself, with
- delusions, imaginations; divided; two parts, into
- delusions, imaginations; wrong; he has done

Taking an inflexible stance so as not to be overwhelmed by the will, thoughts and opinions of others; too inflexible or too flexible:

- aversion; interference
- confusion of mind; conversation agg.
- defiant
- yielding disposition

Violence is still present:

- contradiction; intolerant of; restrain himself, has to, to keep from violence
- kill, desire to

...but not as marked or as impulsive as was the case in Alumina. The vital/emotional self is by now coming more under the control of the rational self. We are now in the established phase of the mental/conceptual self. There is a kind of self-sufficiency and heightened self-esteem:

- egotism, self-esteem; general

Before continuing with some more key remedies in this developmental journey through the periodic table I want to take a pause. I want to do this so that we don't lose sight of the essential developmental process under discussion. There are also one or two other points that are too important to be overlooked any further.

Stages and Phases

Let's just recap on some fundamentals. The human journey is one from unconsciousness through self-consciousness to transpersonal consciousness. That sounds a bit of a bald statement so let's just fill it out a little. Human consciousness rises out of, differentiates itself out of, a primal matrix. The primal matrix has various appellations – nature, universal mother, void, quantum field, to name a few. Everything in nature is of course conscious, but not specifically self-conscious in the human sense. When we talk about unconsciousness and consciousness we are simply using relative terms to describe human consciousness relative to what comes before or after it. Nature herself is an embodiment of consciousness out of which a particularly differentiated form of consciousness, here called human consciousness, arises.

The tragedy is that as human self-consciousness emerges out of the matrix of nature, on its way to transpersonal consciousness of the whole, it disrupts the wholeness of nature, just as the seedpod must burst open and the egg must break. This disruption of nature, especially our own nature, constitutes the foundations of disease.

As far as disease goes, this process of emergence has two aspects. Firstly, emerging self-consciousness forgets the whole of which it is a part and starts to act in its own self-interest. It becomes deluded. The self acquires and maintains illusory beliefs about itself and about the world. The self then acts on the basis of these beliefs. In doing so, and this brings us to the second aspect, it disrupts the rhythms of its own natural foundations. We thus end up with a condition of illusion based on the limited or erroneous sense of self. The wilful activity of this self leads to rhythmic dysfunction; that is to say disturbance of rhythm in the vital functions.

On the big canvas of human evolution the origins of this process can be traced, in broad outline anyway, from the appearance of the first hominids some four million years ago to the present time. On the small canvas of individual development we are born, somewhat whole, but somewhat un-self-conscious, from the relative paradise of our mother's womb. As the self conscious "I" emerges through developmental stages, we forget, deny and repress the instinctual, primal and natural basis of our being.

That's the story of disintegration. What about the story of reintegration? The healthy aim of this process is that self-consciousness should gradually wake up, until eventually it awakens to the whole, which always was and always will be. Ultimately healing means the overcoming of the illusion of separateness that arises in the developmental process. The poets have always reminded us of this circle of life:

> We shall not cease from exploration
> And the end of all our exploring
> Will be to arrive where we started
> And know the place for the first time.
> T. S. Eliot: *Little Gidding* [19]

For this to happen consciousness must expand. From an awareness of physical space, to feeling space, to mental space, to social space, to cultural space and to spiritual space. An awakening to consecutively more inclusive worlds, to consecutively more inclusive holons – the physical world, the vital/emotional world, the mental world, and on to the social holon, the cultural holon and the one-world holon.

With each stage of development, consciousness must give up identification so that it can grow into the next level. The purely physical self must provide the basis for, but also give way to, the more inclusive feeling self. The narcissism of the emotional self must give way to the greater possibilities of the mental self. This in turn must recognise itself as part of a greater whole, the human group, and so on. Thus consciousness must repeatedly undergo birth into a new stage, identification with that stage and the giving up of that stage. We can visualise this cyclical journey through the stages when we look at the periodic table depicted as a spiral (see above).

Each stage develops on the basis of the previous stage. Problems in one's sense of oneself and in one's experience of the world can develop at any stage. Wounds can be sustained at any stage. The demands of the world may well mean that these wounds get repressed. They then form lesions that hamper healthy development. The nearer to the basic matrix that the wound to sense of self occurs the deeper the effect will probably be. For example the body is the carrier of natural instinctive wholeness. If the sense of physical self is traumatised at an early age, then the basis of wholeness and instinctive knowing will be disrupted. (A blow to the body might traumatise the body, but not necessarily the physical sense of self. By contrast physical abuse would traumatise the physical sense of self. It would seriously wound the sense of physical presence at that level. It would wound the foundational sense of "I"). Wounds at the emotional stage can be slight or severe. Severe lesions at these primary levels will have a profound influence on further development.

Once a wound has been sustained it becomes a focus constantly pulling awareness back to itself. It becomes, as it were, a hole in wholeness. For example if you have a carbon issue – that is to say a wound related to the physical sense of self and whether there is going to be enough fuel to survive – then the carbon "issues" will tend to be a sticking point, at any age or at any stage of life. In fact what will happen at later stages of life, when difficulties arise or at times of crisis, is that the carbon "problem" will be reactivated. In times of stress you will feel there is not enough money in the bank, not enough food in the larder and so on. Behind these anxieties lurks a terrible fear that you're not going to make it – an unconscious memory complex from the stage of differentiation of the physical self. Wounds can arise at any stage of development and form the basis of unresolved conflicts, which can remain throughout life as a source of disease.

There is another point that should be made here. Each stage carries developmental difficulties that are normal for that stage.

For example it is normal for the infant to feel that physical safety might be uncertain, or that the loving mother, source of all nourishment and nurture, might not be so loving after all. If a problem of this nature, related to an early stage of development, is recognised, then it is relatively easy to remedy it. Providing the mother is reasonably healthy in her attitude and is doing OK, a well-indicated homœopathic remedy will help the infant to adapt successfully.

However if the problem is habitually reinforced (the mother neglects the child, not just occasionally, but frequently), then the foundations for later difficulties will be laid. If such a problem is not recognised and dealt with, then as further development proceeds it becomes an unconscious problem, undermining the health of the developing personality. One might say that the further away in time one gets from the source of the problem, the more the habits and defences associated with that problem become ingrained. When this happens things become that much more difficult to straighten out.

Of course much will depend on the nature of the problem. For example an adult with anxieties rooted in patterns of unresolved feelings from the age of five or six may be fairly easy to help with homœopathy. However an adult with severe psychological pathologies rooted in the very earliest months of life will present a far greater challenge to the homœopath, and the healing possibilities will be more limited.

Development and cover up

As the self conscious "I" becomes a greater presence in the life of the individual, the foundations are laid for the individual's participation in a world beyond its own. The "I" now has the means to play an active part in the holons of family and society. This brings the opportunity for greater integration. There is however another side to this coin. There is also a greater possibility of becoming more out of touch with one's own nature and instinctive wisdom. Consciousness is often bought at the expense of wholeness. In the remedy Silica, for example, we see splitting and conflict within the self. The mental self struggles to establish itself while at the same time conforming to the expected image.

In order to conform and appear correct, the developing self feels that it is necessary to cover up all that doesn't conform. When we get right down to it, what is it that doesn't conform? It is the instinctive, the animal, the sexual, as well as the playful and spontaneous. It is that which belongs to primal wholeness. When we deny these primal parts of ourselves they don't go away, but hide in the dark, longing for light and acknowledgement, but because denied, on the prowl and threatening. We feel that these parts of ourselves are ugly and that we must keep them from sight. This means we must be on our guard, always in control, in case someone should see the wild and unbridled nature of which we are now so ashamed. We no longer trust ourselves. We no longer trust our own nature. Thus, by projection, we no longer trust others either. We must control and, in extreme cases, become fanatical. This tragic picture is most closely mirrored in the remedy Thuja occidentalis, the tree of life. Here are some characteristic Thuja symptoms:

- confusion of mind; identity, as to his; duality, sensation of
- contemptuous; himself, herself, of
- deceitful, sly
- delusions, imaginations; animals, of; abdomen, in
- delusions, imaginations; criminal, that he is a
- delusions, imaginations; divided; two parts, into
- delusions, imaginations; loved by parents, is not
- delusions, imaginations; ugly, is
- delusions, imaginations; worthless, he is
- delusions, imaginations; wrong; he has done
- fanaticism
- fear; general; self-control, losing
- fear; general; strangers, of
- forsaken feeling; isolation, sensation of
- hide, desire to
- liar
- looked at; cannot bear to be
- religious; affections, general; fanaticism

- secretive
- sensual
- touched; aversion to being [20]

Repression of the instinctual with subsequent guilt, paranoia and cover up speak plainly through these symptoms. There is guilt (done wrong, criminal) and cover up (hiding, secretive) over the natural and instinctual (sensual, animal). Thus the individual ceases to trust himself (ugly, worthless) and indeed becomes untrustworthy (deceitful). The conflict between rational control and the instinctual (divided) means he must stay in control (fear of losing self control, fanatical) in order to keep the outlawed animal nature down.

This is not only a personal tragedy but a collective one as well. Because we learn to deceive ourselves it means we can more easily be deceived. We can be lied to. When we are lied to it means we go along with the general miasm of deceit. This makes it possible for powerful political, industrial and religious groups to lie to themselves and lie to the people. Individuals then go along with the general deceit without too much question.

The phases of the stages

Let's return to the idea of the phases of each stage. Self-consciousness emerges by stages. Each stage is a cycle with a beginning, middle and end. To start with the self must meet the challenge of the new stage. There is desire and hope as well as fear of the unknown. The self then establishes itself at the new stage. As it does this it begins to dis-identify with that stage. It becomes a self that lives within that world (physical, emotional, mental, etc.) but is no longer completely merged with that world. For example at the emotional stage there is eventually a self with emotions, rather than just a world of emotion. Finally the self must dis-identify with that particular stage in preparation for birth into the next stage. Thus each stage of psychological development has a beginning, middle and end. This is the simplest way of dividing up each stage. [21]

Let's just clarify these stages and phases in relation to the periodic table. There are seven stages in the development of the self-conscious "I". These stages correspond, as we discussed above, to the periods of the periodic table.

Scholten calls these periods, series – the Hydrogen series, the Carbon series, and so on.

In the periodic table each series (each one corresponding to a stage in the development of consciousness) is divided into eighteen stages. These are the eighteen vertical columns of the periodic table. The eighteen vertical columns correspond to the maximum number of elements (discounting the elements normally shown as a separate block at the bottom of the periodic table – see Fig. 4.1) in one horizontal row. According to Scholten each series is characterised by a wave motion of ascent, peak and descent. All that's happened is that the basic three steps (beginning, middle, end) of each developmental stage are expanded into the eighteen phases (which Scholten calls stages) of a horizontal row of the periodic table.

We can say then that each stage in the development of consciousness is characterised by a beginning, middle and end. Or, put another way, each series of the periodic table is characterised by eighteen phases in a wave pattern of gradual ascent, peak and decline.

Phases and remedies

Each series (of the periodic table) mirrors a stage of development of consciousness. The individual remedies that make up each series are simply different phases in the ascent, establishment and decline of each series.

Remedies near the beginning of a series belong to beginnings. They reflect the attitudes and anxieties associated with getting started. The remedies in the middle of a series correspond to the establishment of a particular identity.

The remedies at the end of a series are concerned with decline, loss and death. For example, according to Scholten, stage fourteen (in any series) is empty, weak and drained.[22] In stage 15 there can be feelings of loss and death. Stage 17 has the feeling of betrayal, exile and fleeing.[23]

The self can become overly identified with (and thus stuck at) any phase of any stage of development. In other words one can always feel that one has to get started (but can't). Or one always tries to be in control. Or you feel that you inhabit a world of decline and ending, even to the point of destruction, despair and death. Thus normal unfolding is hampered and the dynamic of disease associated with that stage and phase establishes itself.

In the next chapter we'll continue on our elemental journey.

Chapter 5

Homœopathic Correspondences
(continued)

Periodic Table (continued)

Let's continue the developmental journey through the spiral of life.

Mental/conceptual stage (continued)
Phosphorus

The symptoms of Phosphorus are numerous and well known. Let's summarise. Sympathetic; needs company; fears, of being alone, darkness, twilight and so on; can go to the opposite polarity (of sympathy and company), namely in-difference, to family, to loved ones.

What about the "signature" of Phosphorus? The word Phosphorus is from the Greek, meaning "bearer of light." In Latin this is "Lucifer."

Phosphorus burns at room temperature with a cold flame. In fact it is so inflammable that it has to be kept under water (a very thirsty remedy!). In the body it is most concentrated in two systems: in the bones (in the form of Calcium phosphate), and in the brain and central nervous system.

Taking this well-known symptom picture, together with these "signatures", what can we say about the remedy in relation to the mental conceptual stage of development?

Phosphorus is the light-bearer. The element is found particularly in the brain and nervous system. Surely we are here in the realm of the "light of reason?"

We are in the realm of awareness, the realm of cognition. We might say that the Phosphorus pathology rests on an imbalance of awareness. There is, as it were, too much awareness. The Phosphorus individual is overwhelmed by impressions and cannot maintain "awareness boundaries." Impressions from the surroundings can't be kept out. There is clairvoyance (awareness beyond the boundaries of normal time); sympathy (taking on the feelings and impressions of another); great tendency to start; oversensitive to external impressions; quickly prostrated by unpleasant impressions; anxiety for others. In short the Phosphorus subject is affectionate, sympathetic, open, impressionable, clairvoyant.

This sensitivity isn't only to external impressions. Images from the unconscious invade awareness. There is "fearfulness, as if something were creeping out of every corner" and "fear of imaginary things."[1] It is as though too much is entering awareness from both within and without.

Phosphorus also fears that which represents the dimming of the light of awareness;[2] namely darkness, twilight. They also need company and fear being alone, as though darkness and isolation would overwhelm them.

In the mental/conceptual stage of development the self begins to develop the faculties of reason and logic. The light of consciousness begins to shine forth. As far as the periodic table goes this development becomes possible in the third series, the series that corresponds to the psychological "I" (emotional and mental stages of development). According to Scholten this series is concerned with relationships. It is to do with "I" and "other." From this basis flow the other themes of the series – communication, language and learning.

It is in relationship to others that we develop a sense of "I." Phosphorus has great awareness of others. They also feel alone with a great need for company, contact and reassurance.

The Phosphorus person can also be fascinated with themselves. Catherine Coulter writes, "He considers himself more sensitive and refined, more intuitive, more entertaining, more gifted, more spiritual than others. He can be quite fascinated with himself and view his person as the centre around which others revolve, or as a latter-day Prometheus whose talents enrich mankind like the fire stolen from heaven."[3] It is as though he believes himself to be the light, rather than the bearer of light:

- delusions, imaginations; distinguished
- delusions, imaginations; great person, is

- delusions, imaginations; lifted up, he or she is
- delusions, imaginations; noble person, he is a
- delusions, imaginations; rank, he is a person of
- delusions, imaginations; wealth, of

An elevated sense of self, who feels above the every day world. As with its neighbours, Silica and Sulphur, there is an element of ego here. These remedies are concerned with identity and self-image (corresponding with the mental/conceptual stage of development). The pathology of these remedies (and of this stage of development) is excessive self-centredness.

If man is the bearer of the light of awareness and reason in the world of nature, then this is surely a double-edged sword.

In the myth of Lucifer, the angel is thrown out of heaven (he falls from heaven) by an angry God for his rebelliousness against God. He had claimed that "I will ascend above the heights of the clouds, I will be like the most high." [4] We might say that the lesson of the Phosphorus phase of development is that Phosphorus is *the light bearer and not the light itself.*

Moving one step further we come to Sulphur

Sulphur

Sulphur is more down to earth and more obviously selfish than Phosphorus. It is the embodiment of spirit, as heat. It is fire rather than light. It is as though, with Sulphur, the heat of the Sun takes up residence in the flesh. There are said to be two basic types, the philosopher, with his ungrounded flights of fancy, and the more earthy practical idealist.[5]

At this stage we encounter the awakening of the awareness that "I am I." This is the ego as a burning ember of the true Self. Thus in the pathology of this phase of mental/conceptual development the issue is ego, and in extremis, nothing but ego.

The developing sense of self (the ego as spark of the true Self) thrives when it is bathed in the warmth of admiration. If there has been a lack of this warming admiration in the development of one who particularly needs it (who has susceptibility in this direction), then the ego will crave it, and development will be stuck at this stage:

- ailments from; reputation, from loss of
- ailments from; scorn, being scorned
- delusions, imaginations; disgraced; she is
- desires; beautiful things, finery
- flattery; gives everything, when flattered

This leads to a struggle to succeed, in order to get the recognition and status they feel they lack:

- ailments from; business; failure
- delusions, imaginations; failure, he is a
- despair; social position, of
- fear; general; failure, of

There arises a kind of deluded egotism that cannot see beyond itself. There is deluded self-satisfaction. (Sulphur belongs to column 16. Among the themes given by Scholten for this stage are loss, decay, laziness and neglect.) There is a kind of delusion of being in paradise, when you're actually in shit! (Sulphur can be excessively sensitive to their own body odour, or completely disinterested in cleanliness):

- cheerfulness, gaiety, happiness; general; foolish, and
- delusions, imaginations; abundance of everything, she has an
- delusions, imaginations; beautiful, wonderful; rags are, even
- delusions, imaginations; great person, is
- egotism, self-esteem; general
- foolish behaviour; happiness and pride

Eventually they no longer care about what others think. They are self-satisfied in their own greatness, even if nobody else sees it:

- business; neglects his
- dirtiness; general
- indifference, apathy; appearance, about personal
- indifference, apathy; business affairs, to

- indifference, apathy; welfare of others, to
- indolence; aversion to work

As an archetype, Sulphur gives the ability to question and understand (theorising, philosophising). The pathology of the Sulphur archetype is the self's conviction of its own greatness and concomitant need for appreciation.

Let's move on now to the rule/role stage of development.

Rule/role mind

This stage of development ushers in an awareness of the immediate group, a capacity to take care of the immediate group and an awareness of the rules and roles that constitute the cohesion of the group. This stage corresponds to the fourth period. Here are some of the key words that Scholten gives for this period: task, work, duty, skill, order, rules, control, criticised, failure, guilt, police.[6] According to Scholten the area of awareness is the village. In the rule/role stage of development the self becomes more sociocentric, developing an awareness of the immediate group. Let's turn to the first major remedy of the fourth period, Kali carbonicum.

Kali carbonicum

Here are some key words for the Kali group of remedies, as understood by Scholten – principles, duty, work, family. In Vermeulen we read (based on the teachings of George Vithoulkas), "Common traits of all Kali's: conservative, regular, proper, down to earth. 'Lot of emphasis on morality and what is right, what is wrong. Black and white issues.' "

"Strong mental control. Fear of losing control … dogmatic … strong sense of duty." [7]

These clinical observations speak for themselves. We're in the rule/role stage of development. In this stage awareness expands beyond the boundaries of "I", to an awareness of the immediate group. Sankaran writes, "The main theme of Kali carbonicum is the vital fear and reactivity (carbon) that is seen when a person lacks the support of a family or group (kali)." [8]

So, the themes of work, duty, morals and family come together in Kali carbonicum. In short, rules, roles and an expansion of awareness to include the group. It is in the family that the rules and roles that form the basis of social cohesion are learnt. The emphasis on family by one homœopathic observer and the emphasis on morals by another are really two views of one phenomenon. (The third series of the periodic table is also concerned with the family, but in the sense of relationships, not rules and roles).

There is vital fear and need for support:

- carried; desires to be
- fear; general; alone, of being
- fear; general; death, of; alone, when
- fear; general; disease, of; impending
- fear; general; poverty

However there is also aversion to the group:

- aversion; family members, to
- misanthropy

Self or group? This produces conflict:

- anarchist (particularly Causticum, another kali salt)
- antagonism; herself, with
- capriciousness
- company; desire for; alone, agg. while
- company; desire for; treats them outrageously, yet
- desires; change, always
- fear; general; alone, of being; desire of being alone, but
- quarrelsome, scolding; family, with his or her
- self-control; want of

Kali carbonicum thus expresses the struggle of the early phases of the rule/role stage of consciousness. It has the survival fears of carbon coupled with a need to follow the rules and receive the protection of the group.

Ferrum

The element lies in column 8 of the fourth series. Iron has an affinity with the circulation. The homœopathic picture is characterised by flushing, haemorrhages, anaemia and other circulatory disorders. Iron is the carrier. Its presence in haemoglobin enables the carrying of oxygen. Iron is thus essential to combustion. It makes us think of red blood and muscle power; of the power to exercise the will; of having an iron will.

When we think of the industrial revolution we think of muscle power. We think of ships, trains, iron bridges and buildings – power to make things, move things and shape the world. Since then iron and steel have been essential to the world of manufacturing. Physically we are reliant on steel.

The industrial age coincided with the height of the most extensive empire the world has ever seen. The establishment and protection of trading routes was often an important factor in the expansion of the British Empire.

The Iron Age itself (beginning around 1250 B.C.) was characterised more than anything by the figure of the warrior and a culture of war and conquest. The laying waste of cities and populations became the norm.[9]

How can we summarise all this? It makes us think of will and the imposition of order – either fighting against others imposing their will on you, or forcing your will on others. Sankaran suggests that the main feeling in Ferrum is being compelled to do something against one's wishes (by parents), and fighting against this.[10]

Others force their will on you, or you force your will on others:

- anger, irascibility; general; contradiction, from
- contradict, disposition to
- delusions, imaginations; war, being at
- dictatorial, domineering, dogmatic, despotic
- disputatious

Force of will (dictatorial) or being imposed upon by the will of another (contradiction). Force must be used to establish your will in a world of rules and impositions.

Interestingly the ancients understood iron to be the metal of the planet Mars, the planet of war and conquest.

Arsenicum album

Arsenic lies in column 15 of the fourth series. We would therefore expect to find symptoms associated with loss (stage 15) of safety and security within the group (fourth series). As a remedy Arsenicum album, the white oxide of arsenic is known for a compulsive need for order:

- compulsive disorders; ritualistic
- conscientious about trifles
- fastidious
- rest; cannot, when things are not in proper place

There is terrific anxiety if they sense "disorder" in their own health:

- anxiety; health, about; despair of getting well

The obsessive need for order compensates a feeling of insecurity. They no longer feel safe within the group. Their security within the group is deeply threatened:

- ailments from; discords between; relatives, friends
- anxiety; health, about; relatives, of
- anxiety; others, for
- begging, entreating
- carried; desires to be
- company; desire for; alone, agg. while
- delusions, imaginations; starve; family will
- fear; general; alone, of being
- fear; general; death, of; alone, when
- forsaken feeling; beloved by his parents, wife, friends, feels is not being
- helplessness, feeling of

Why should they feel so insecure in the group? Because they have a guilty conscience. They actually have, or imagine they have, broken the rules of the group on which they feel themselves to be dependent:

- anxiety; conscience, of
- anxiety; salvation, about
- delusions, imaginations; murdered; someone, he has
- delusions, imaginations; offended people, that he has
- fear; general; arrested, of being

Thus they try to stick to the rules even harder:

- anxiety; salvation, about; scruples, excessive religious
- anxiety; duty, as if he had not done his

Or they start to see the group as a threat. He has broken the rules and now the group is out to get him. The group on which he depended, which once gave him security, now becomes a threat to his safety:

- company; desire for; alone, agg. while; yet fear of people
- delusions, imaginations; injury; receive, will
- delusions, imaginations; murder; conspiring to murder him, others are
- delusions, imaginations; thieve, thieves, robbers, robbing; sees; night
- delusions, imaginations; watched, that she is being
- fear; general; murdered, of being
- fear; general; robbers, of
- hide, desire to; fear, from
- suspiciousness, mistrustfulness

In desperation he turns against the group:

- kill, desire to
- kill, desire to; loved ones

Or himself:

- suicidal disposition; hanging, by (the traditional capital punishment for major crime)

Arsenicum represents a phase in which there is obsession with order for fear of losing the protective security of the group.

(Scholten maintains that the Arsenicum album picture is partly due to the fact that it is an oxide. He suggests that the oxygen picture – carbon series, stage 16 – revolves around selfishly living on, and thus using up, resources and possessions.)

Let's move now to the formal reflexive stage.

Formal-reflexive stage

To continue on the path of self-development the individual must become "post-conventional".[11] You learn to think and imagine for yourself. There is a need to think in ways that are not simply defined by society's rules and roles. When individuals can dream their own dreams and think their own thoughts, then understanding, art and teaching become possible. The formal-reflexive stage corresponds to the fifth period. Scholten calls this period the Silver series. Here are some of the key words he gives for this series: creation; inspiration; ideas; culture; admiration; aesthetics; art; science; mysticism; performance; voice; hearing.[12] Here we are in the realm of ideas, art, performance, understanding and teaching.

We'll go directly to Palladium as the first well known remedy that we come to in the fifth series.

Palladium

With Palladium we are in the middle (stage 10) of the Silver series (corresponding to the establishment phase of the formal reflexive developmental stage).

The word Palladium comes from the Greek, *palladion*, meaning a sacred image or statue. A Palladium was a sacred image or statue of the goddess Pallas Athene, or one made by her. There were several such images, known collectively as palladia. It is told that the Palladium was sent by Zeus to Dardanus, the founder of Troy. It was believed that the city could not be taken as long as it possessed the Palladium.[13]

So a Palladium was a sacred image of Pallas Athene. What about the goddess herself? She is the Greek goddess of wisdom and crafts. She also presided over battle strategy in wartime. She was a protector of cities, patron of military forces and goddess of weavers, goldsmiths, potters and dressmakers.

Her bird was the owl – the one who sees in the dark. Her birth was remarkable. She sprang from Zeus's head as a full-grown woman, wearing flashing gold armour, with a sharp spear in one hand, emitting a mighty war cry.

Without turning to the symptomology of the metal yet, what might we say based upon the evidence of the mythological complex from which the metal's name derives? Clearly we are in the realm of imagination and art – the sacred image of the goddess of art and culture. The notion that art could be anything other than sacred was unthinkable in the ancient world. Thus we are in the world of sacred art. What does this mean? Because all true art – as well as philosophy and science – attempts to reach beyond the mundane to the realm of creative imagination that stands behind manifest reality, it is in its essence sacred. The artist attempts to peer into the darkness to give expression and form to the informing dynamics and images of the world of imagination. All true artists, philosophers and scientists must attempt to do this. Without this capacity, no art, no understanding and no wisdom.

Athene herself was born fully armed from Zeus' head. She represents the birth of ideas.

Let's now turn to the symptoms of Palladium:

- ailments from; egotism
- ailments from; honour, wounded
- contemptuous
- delusions, imaginations; appreciated, that she is not
- delusions, imaginations; insulted, he or she is
- delusions, imaginations; neglected; he is
- delusions, imaginations; tall, taller; he is
- egotism, self-esteem; general
- flattery; desires
- forsaken feeling
- haughty; wounded, wishes to be flattered
- longing for; good opinion of others
- social; position, concerned about

What does this tell us? The person who needs this remedy wants flattery and the good opinion of others. The feeling is "admire me, I am so special and precious." She "keeps up brightly in company", and her pride is easily wounded.[14] Curiously it is traditionally a woman's remedy (the goddess) with a special affinity for the ovaries (creative). They feel themselves to be special and above others (as though they themselves were an image of the divine). If she is not flattered, she feels insulted or neglected, as though her true worth is not being recognised.

What can we make of all this in the light of the mythology surrounding Palladium as both sacred image and metal? In the formal reflexive stage of development the individual starts to imagine. When you can imagine, there is the possibility of creativity and understanding. We might say that the function of art, science, and teaching is to reflect a higher understanding.

The artist/scientist attempts to give expression to the archetypal world of images and ideas. It is necessary for a culture to maintain its connection with this creative world. If a culture fails to maintain its connection with this inner world through its artists, poets, writers, scientists, experimenters and dreamers, it loses inspiration. It collapses from within (as long as Troy had the Palladium, the city could not be taken).

In healthy development the Palladium phase represents the summation of the establishment of the formal reflexive stage of consciousness, with its capacity for independent thinking and dreaming. We could say that in the pathology of this stage of development, the individual wants others to reflect back to them, to their ego, wonder and appreciation rather than they themselves reflecting the wonder of the sacred world of the imagination.

This notion of image and reflection will become apparent in a slightly different way in the next metal, Argentum metallicum.

Argentum metallicum
With silver we are in the realm of image, reflection and the capacity to be a "conductor" – of light, of sound, of energy. Let's look at the signature.

The use of silver in mirrors attests to its reflective capacity. The light sensitivity and capacity to hold an image of photographic paper is due to silver salts. Bells and musical instruments made of silver have the sweetest tones. Silver is the best conductor (better than copper) of heat and electricity.

It is as though the metal offers little resistance to the channelling of image, sound or energy. We might say then that the "silver function" gives the human being the ability to "channel" and thus give form to the imaginational realm. The alchemists of the past held that silver was the metal of the moon.

But (like Palladium) the individual becomes concerned with their own ability to perform. They feel a need to be valued (like the precious metal). The capacity to channel is mixed up with the stress arising from the need for admiration and the pressure to perform. The capacity to sing, speak or write brings with it the need to be admired. In this sense the performer gets caught up in bathing in reflected glory. They can lose sight of the fact that their function is to give form to the invisible world of ideas, sound and imagination. With Argentum we are moving into the decline of the Silver series (stage 11). Thus fear of failure and anxiety about performance becomes that much greater, as particularly demonstrated in Argentum nitricum. Sankaran puts it well, "The Argentum metallicum situation is one where the person has to perform intellectually and express himself through speech, singing, writing, etc., and also has to defend himself by intellect, speech and words." [15]

Loss of voice in speakers and singers is a typical Argentum pathology. There is also loss of control in mind and nervous system. "Limbs feel powerless." "Loss of mental power." [16] They feel a need to perform perfectly. This requires ability and control of your faculties. The strain of performance and control is too much. As with so much pathology, healing involves learning to trust the process rather than control the process.

Stannum

Stannum (tin) has atomic number 50, and stands well into the decline of the fifth series (corresponding to the decline of the formal-reflexive stage):

• delusions, imaginations; afternoon, that it is always

The keyword for Stannum is emptiness. They feel empty of ideas and inspiration: [17]

• concentration; difficult; attempting to, on; vacant feeling, has a
• emptiness of the mind, sensation of

They are just going through the motions of inspiration and creativity:

- busy; fruitlessly
- muttering; absurd things

As though they are living in the past:

- sentimental

and feel no longer admired:

- ailments from; admonition; kindly
- sensitive, oversensitive; general; others say about her, what

They can no longer find the inspiration:

- persists in nothing

The feeling of inner emptiness brings about a desperate feeling similar to that found in Arsenicum:

- begging, entreating
- carried; desires to be

The chest is the place of "inspiration". They are empty of "inspiration":

- voice; weak; talking, after
- chest; weakness; general; talking, when
- chest; empty sensation

Stannum has the curious symptom (only remedy in rubric, also in bold type):

- respiration; difficult; dressing, while

Can we make any sense of this symptom? Putting clothes on is connected with presenting an image to the world. Dressing also often involves mirrors. With the decline of inner worth, outer image becomes more important (Scholten says about Stannum: formal presentation of yourself). The stress of having to maintain this image produces a difficulty in breathing.

Stannum is about the pathology of emptiness. It might also be about the opportunity of emptiness. When there is inward emptiness creative inspiration and ideas can flow through the artist, teacher or thinker, thus finding form in the human world.

The Vision-logic stage

This stage brings a higher and wider perspective. At this stage we reach the possibility of inner integration. The self is no longer particularly identified with body or mind. The self now begins to transcend both mind and body. There is a broader perspective in which thinking, feeling and doing can be integrated. There is greater awareness of the whole.

Seeing the whole brings with it responsibility for the whole. Scholten notes that vision and vision problems are connected with the Gold series, the series that corresponds to this stage of development.[18] Individuals who need remedies from this series can hold (or aspire to hold) positions of power, authority and responsibility.

True authority holds the parts together in an integrated whole. It is the centre point, like the sun in the solar system, the king in the state, or the heart in the body.

However, inner power and integration are not to be confused with the kind of power and domination a person exercises *over* themselves or others. Authorship and integration are the positive expression of this stage. Domination is the negative expression.

This stage corresponds with the sixth period. Among the key ideas given by Scholten for the Gold series are: king, leadership, management; responsibility for a larger whole (such as a company or nation); representative of the divine will on Earth; power, dictatorship; isolation; serious, heavy; failure.[19]

Platina

Platinum stands in the middle (column 10) of the sixth series. The symptoms of Platina are well known. They centre around pride, superiority and the need to be regarded as the best, the highest and the most valuable. They suffer from the effects of scorn, dishonour and failed ambition.

They have the capacity for the higher perspective:

- delusions, imaginations; tall, taller; he is

but feel superior:

- contemptuous; everything, of
- delusions, imaginations; humility and lowness of others, while he is great

or inferior, as though their true value is not recognised:

- ailments from; scorn, being scorned
- delusions, imaginations; appreciated, that she is not

Their superior position makes them feel isolated and cut off:

- delusions, imaginations; strange; land, in a

Sankaran sums it up like this, "Everything about her is rare, valuable, spiritual, intellectual. Now she feels big inside. At the same time, being so special and rare, she feels left out in a world of ordinary people – she cannot mix or mingle with them. She cannot form relationships with other people just as the noble metal platinum cannot easily form a compound. So there is a feeling of loneliness, of isolation – a feeling of being the 'Queen', yet of being alone." [20]

She is contemptuous of everything "lowly" including her own "lower nature." He or she has a strong sexual nature (the remedy is known for nymphomania), which is in conflict with a lofty intellectual or spiritual position:

- religious; affections, general; alternating with sexual excitement
- religious; affections, general; horror of the opposite sex

In this remedy, in common with other remedies of the series, we see a lofty position in life together with a more destructive pathology. Threats to her greatness must be removed:

- delusions, imaginations; enemy; everyone is an
- kill, desire to; knife; sight of a, at
- kill, desire to; loved ones

Aurum metallicum

Gold is the most precious of metals. It is called a noble metal because it is extremely resistant to chemical action. A heavy metal (atomic number 79), and yet can be beaten to translucent fineness in the form of gold leaf. Since ancient times its beauty and lustre has been seen as the expression on Earth of something otherworldly. It was seen as a manifestation of the Sun and of the divine. The alchemists sought the gold – that is the incorruptible divinity – within themselves.

But the history of gold is also a story of corruption. I'll extract from Wilhelm Pelikan's excellent essay on gold. "In ancient times gold served only cultic purposes; it belonged to the priest-king, who kept it in trust for the sun-god … After the fall of Persia all the gold of the ancient world streamed into the hands of one man, Alexander the Great. He was one of the first who stood entirely by the strength of his own personality. He was also the first to adorn gold coins with a human image, his own. He inaugurated a redistribution of gold throughout the then known world. After his death it flowed into all parts."[21]

This is the story of the usurping of divine power and radiance by the ego. The ego identifies with a power beyond itself, the power and radiance of life. It is this identification by the ego with a power beyond itself that brings about corruption. The use and abuse of power by the ego brings about corruption. When the ego attempts to hold what cannot be held, then it must hasten destruction of self and others. Thus the well-known maxim, "power corrupts, and absolute power corrupts absolutely." Gold is known for deeply destructive pathologies.

Let's now turn to the remedy. The picture is one of heavy responsibility and sense of duty. "He demands of himself industry and responsibility, conscientiousness and duty of the highest degree, uncompromising princi-ples or goals that are beyond the possible." [22] He is the leader charged with responsibility for family, company, nation. He takes that heavy responsibility seriously. He is plagued by feelings of having failed (stage 11) in his duty, of having failed his flock (sixth series). He feels he has let himself or others down. Thus he is "oversensitive to contradiction; resulting in explosive fits of anger and violence." [23] He holds on to power and responsibility.[24] As long as he can carry this great responsibility he remains reasonably intact. However if he fails, or feels that he is failing, then the result is the well-known Aurum pathology – self-condemnation and eventually a desire to die.

It is as though he feels himself to be the representative of the divine on Earth. He takes that onerous calling very seriously, and thus, in his hour of darkness he turns to God; Aurum is a prominent remedy in the rubric "pray-ing." In his final hour of desperation, as if in an effort to compensate for his untenable position of lofty responsibility and isolation, he throws himself from a high place. After all, the thought of suicide has often brought a sense of peace.

Mercury
Mercury is one of the most destructively poisonous of substances. It destroys tissues, the nervous system and the mind. In this it is similar to the disease syphilis, for which it was the main remedy (various compounds of mercury, in both allopathic and homœopathic medicine).

Let's look briefly at its signature. Despite being a heavy metal (atomic number 80), which is twice as dense as iron and fourteen times as heavy as water, it is a liquid. It is easily scattered into droplets due to a lack of inner cohesion. And yet it comes back together again just as easily. Each drop is also able to round itself out and close its form. It seems to both have and lack cohesion.

Its mutable nature is also revealed in the fact that it is extremely reactive to temperature and atmospheric changes (thermometers, barometers). As a metal it is similar to the noble metals (gold, platinum, etc.) in that it is imper-vious to such environmental influences as dampness and air.[25]

In the organism Mercury destroys tissues. Ulceration and necrosis are its hallmarks. In the laboratory the metal dissolves other metals, such as gold, silver and zinc, to make amalgams.

How can we summarise this – noble, cohesive, while at the same time being unstable, changeable, incohesive and destructive (dissolving).

The Gold series (corresponding to the vision-logic stage of development) is concerned with power, control and responsibility. With Mercurius (column 12) we are entering the phase of decline or destruction of power. It is a remedy associated with dictators and the overthrow of dictators. Sankaran sums up the picture like this:

"The main feeling in Mercurius is that of being dominated, suppressed or contradicted by an extremely dictatorial authority. The only solution in such a situation is to either get away from or revolt against this domination. The Mercurius person feels viciously attacked on all sides. He has the delusion that he is surrounded by enemies, that everyone around is an enemy and he has to fight his way out. This is a desperate situation that necessitates a desperate reaction. And so with Mercurius as with other syphilitic remedies, the accent is on destruction, either of himself or others. While on the one hand he feels dominated and defies authority, on the other he can become quite dictatorial himself." [26]

On the world stage he is the dictator that must keep his power and hold the crumbling empire together whatever the cruelty and suppression involved. Or he is the anarchist that must destroy the harsh rule of the dictator. Quite possibly he started as the former (anarchist) and became the latter (dictator).

Everything must decline and decay. The decline of power leads to ruthless dictatorship and corruption.

Heavy metals, death and spirituality

With the heavy metals Platina and Aurum we reach the pinnacle of the development of personal self-consciousness. They lie in the middle of the sixth series and correspond to the middle phase of the vision-logic stage of development (Platina at the height, "I am the summit" – Aurum already going into decline, "holding onto responsibility and warding off failure").[27] At this stage the mature self has the view from the heights. These individuals are, as it were, at the top of the mountain. They have reached the pinnacle of achievement, either in terms of personal development or in terms of worldly achievement, or both. (The early remedies in this series represent the feelings of someone faced with the challenge of climbing the mountain, of scaling the heights of power and responsibility. For example Baryta is like a handicapped person who has to climb a mountain.) [28]

Mountaintops have also, since ancient times, been places where people went to commune with the divine. Thus these metals are near the divine. They stand on the brink of the transpersonal (praying, religious affections, etc.). However, in their pathology they look down from the heights but have not yet learned to look up into the beyond from whence their true power and calling comes. They think it's all down to them, and, in thinking that, their feeling of aloneness and isolation is further exacerbated.

Being at the height of ego development they suffer from the most destructive of ego pathologies. They have reached, or strive to reach, the height of worldly achievement. They are charged with great responsibilities. And thus in their failure they stand to lose – everything! Pathology at this level is characterised by destruction, despair, hatred, paranoia and death.

The point is they have reached the stage where the ego can no longer sort it out. These metals represent the final desperate illusions, trials and battles of the personal self. For healing to happen they must realise that their power is not theirs. It manifests through them. If they don't realise the need for ego death consciously, then they will try and kill something else – either themselves or others; either that or the processes of death will take hold of their bodily tissues.

Mercury offers us a clue as to the way out here. The metal was recognised by the alchemists to be an earthly representative of the god Mercury, known to the Greeks as Hermes. Mercury was god of thieves and merchants, reminding us that we are in the realm, in common with the other heavy metals, of value, wealth, power and corruption. However, Hermes (the Greek incarnation of the god Mercury) was also a psychopomp, which means that he was the guide of souls to the underworld.

When the personal self reaches its maximum potential it must accept a higher power than itself, accept transformation or undergo the hell of its own destruction. Going beyond the personal self means facing a kind of death – a death of all you falsely believed yourself to be; death of the illusions (to which the ego clings) of importance and separation. It means to journey in your own underworld to face your own demons and ancestral pathologies. This is indeed the darkness before the dawn. Mercury the remedy stands for destruction of earthly authority, be it an internal one (ego) or an external one (dictator). Hermes the psychopomp guides you into the realm of death so that you might embrace the next stage of development – birth into the true Self – in which you must go beyond ego and personal inclinations. But first we must negotiate the realm of the radioactive metals.

The transpersonal

The stages of the transpersonal, as we have seen, represent stages of development beyond the personal self. There is a move from self-centredness (with a small "s") to being centred in the Self (with a capital "S"). The transpersonal Self is no longer personal. It embraces – transcends and includes – the personal, but is itself beyond the personal. As we saw, Wilber, based on the teachings of the great mystics of both East and West, delineates four stages of the transpersonal. In the first there is union with nature. This is a conscious union, not an unconscious symbiosis, as exists at developmental stages zero. In the second there is union with the deity, a sacred marriage of spirit and soul. In the third, the formless, there is realisation of the one Self, the Self that is the Self of all creation. Consciousness is now identified with the void, with the ground from which all manifestation arises; the changeless, formless Self out of which space, time and all creation are born. In the final stage all notions of subject and object, Seer and Seen is dissolved. There is only pure, undifferentiated, unbroken consciousness.

I don't want to dwell too much on these stages, partly because of the inadequacy of words to describe something that is beyond words. However, what might be the signs that the self is beginning to be absorbed into the Transpersonal realm? Compassion for self and others. The capacity to attend to what is going on in and around you with care and non-judgement. An ability to be led by the prompting of wise Nature in her presence as body sensation, feeling and intuition. A greater capacity to live with the opposites within oneself – mind and body; masculine and feminine; action and non-action; community and aloneness. A sense of sureness that is not based on ego, rather it is a resting and certainty in the succour of the Self.

Above all, however, if one is to cross the threshold from the personal to the transpersonal one must be prepared to undergo death, not once, but repeatedly. By this I mean ego death: an ongoing stripping away of false images, feelings and ideas about yourself and the world. Only thus can the true Self shine forth.

This stripping is often painful because the personal self likes to cling to what it has and what it knows. Thus we have to learn to die many times over. Death is always a descent. The ego likes to ascend to lofty heights of light and self-importance. The soul's journey however is into the underworld in order to undergo death and rebirth. This takes us into the realm of the radioactive metals.

The radioactive metals

These belong mainly to the elements of the seventh series starting with Francium at atomic number 87 and ending (currently) with Meitnerium at 109. Radioactive atoms emit different kinds of particles due to the disintegration of the nucleus of the atom. These emissions are extremely destructive to human health. They cause cancer and genetic mutations.

Let's look at signatures. The nucleus of a radioactive element is disintegrating. Thus with the Uranium series (seventh period) we are, from a developmental point of view, in the realm of disintegration. What might this mean? Disintegration of what? One acquires, in the course of development, a "nucleus" of ideas, images, beliefs, feelings and patterns of reaction. This nucleus defines how you think, feel and behave in the world. It's what holds you together. However, as we've seen, this nucleus can be a false self, concealing the source of creation and light that is your true Self.

The true Self must, and can only, shine forth. If it is prevented then it becomes a kind of nuclear destruction, appearing in the form of pathologies such as cancer or psychosis. However, if one is to be born into your true Self, then the old nucleus must, so to speak, disintegrate.

Breakdown of the normal personality can be very pathological or very transformative. Breakdown and breakthrough can look similar. The former is a pathological disintegration of the personality. The latter is the death that ushers in spiritual rebirth.

When we think of the radioactive metals and of radiation we of course also think of cancer. Cancer is a breakdown of physical cohesion. Under complaints for the Uranium series Scholten lists cancer, AIDS, genetic defects and leukaemia.[29]

In the myths of the past, the death of the old personality and the birth of the true Self were imagined as an underworld journey in which the hero typically undergoes such trials as battling with a dragon, descent into a whale's belly, or dismemberment. At the nadir of this journey the hero finds his sacred bride, steals a life-giving elixir, and so on. This leads to a return or a resurrection.[30] In the shamanic initiations of the past the shaman also was required to undergo the death of the "ordinary" personality, in order that he might be initiated into the reality of the transpersonal world. This death was understood as a dismemberment at the hands of spirits.[31]

The developmental stage that corresponds to the Uranium series is the threshold and entry into the more inclusive order of the transpersonal levels. Of course the higher levels of the transpersonal, the formless and the non-dual, don't correspond to a series of the periodic table at all. These stages are beyond form. Here the self is identified with the void – the quantum field – out of which the elements arise in the first place.

Little is known homœopathically of the radioactive metals. Radium bromatum has a reasonably developed picture, although it has been used mainly for the effects of radiotherapy. Uranium nitricum has a small picture. Plutonium nitricum has had a full Hahnemannian proving by Jeremy Sherr.[32] Further provings are taking place, and clinical work has been done with some of the metals on the basis of Scholten's indications.[33] However I would suggest, based on what is so far known, that their therapeutic domain is the process of disintegration discussed above. The signature of some of the metals is instructive.

Radium produces terrible radiation burns.

Uranium is named after Uranus, the sky god who united with his mother, Gaia, who thence gave birth to the Titans as well as other giants and monsters such as the one-eyed Cyclopes. Uranus was so horrified with the offspring (as well he might be considering the history of the twentieth century) that he shut them up in the depths of the Earth.

Neptunium is named after Neptune, or Poseidon, the god of the ocean. He could cause tempest and raging seas as well as instantly calm storms.

Plutonium is named after the god Pluto or Hades. He is the god of the underworld, the "invisible one" and god of riches. He presides over the underworld and the shades of the dead. He is unseen and rarely leaves the underworld. His most notable sortie to the daylight world was to abduct and rape Persephone.

It is clear from these allusions that we are below, in the world of unconscious forces, of darkness and death. This is the realm, the myths tell us, that must be traversed if we are to awaken to our true Self and true calling in life.

Let's turn to Plutonium because we have Sherr's proving and Scholten's commentary. These are some of the themes that emerged in the events, feelings and dreams of the proving. Breaking glass; depression and isolation; dark and empty; tall/elongated, looking down from a great height; being half human and half animal; feeling like a cave man or an amoeba in the sea; the legacy of past generations; dreams of the underworld. Among the themes given by Scholten (based on data from Sherr's proving) are: prehistory and primitive instincts; genetic history and mutations (half human, half animal); magic and out of the body experiences; broken glass.[34]

This represents going back to the roots of what you are. Going back to your genetic inheritance that you might know and thus dis-identify with the sins of the forefathers. And there you find at the nadir of matter, on the shores of the endless mystery of emptiness, that you are Shiva, the creator and the destroyer, and that the divine fire that burns within all manifestation is at once the creator of form and destroyer of form. You negotiate the twists and turns of your genetic inheritance to find the ultimate secret of death and life, death in life and life in death. This is the gateway to the transpersonal realm. Among the key ideas given by Scholten for the Uranium series are: the magus or shaman, intuition, and old age.

Developmental Worlds

We have considered the developmental stages through which self-consciousness emerges. At each stage the self is faced with the challenges of growing into the next stage. It has to establish itself at each consecutive stage (as a physical self, an emotional self, and so on). In order to continue to grow, the self then has to sacrifice its identity with that stage. It has to give something up. If it is able to do this successfully then it retains the capabilities and functions of that stage (an emotional life for example), but is able also to move beyond complete rulership by that stage. This involves a dis-identification.

For example, if you are only an emotional self there is no emotional free-dom. You are identified with the emotional world. It is only when a further stage of development can emerge (the mental/conceptual), with its capacity for a more inclusive sphere of awareness, that some freedom from unconscious immersion in the currents of the emotional world becomes possible. When we talk about or analyse our feelings we are in fact doing so from the more eman-cipated perspective of a higher stage of development. We are able to under-stand our feelings *because* we are outside them and relatively free of them.

We can picture each stage as surrounding and containing the previous stages (like concentric spheres). Thus the self is first of all a physical self and then a physical *and* emotional self, then a physical self *and* emotional self *and* mental self, and so on. Thus at each stage greater depth is added. At any stage of development you have the previous stages within you. Health depends on the way of being and the worldview that is characteristic of each

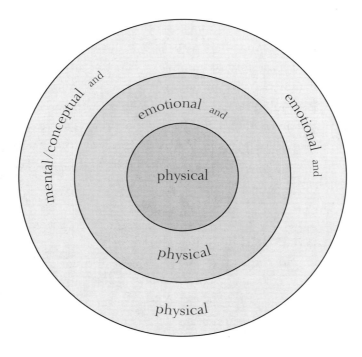

Fig. 5.1 Developmental stages as concentric spheres

The emotional sphere transcends and includes the physiosphere. The mental/conceptual sphere transcends and includes the emotional sphere and physiosphere.

previous stage being successfully integrated into your wholeness. What tends to happen, as we have seen, is that the self lives in a particular sphere of reality (the mental/conceptual for example), and denies or represses other levels. This happens especially when there is trauma or pain at a previous level (the emotional for example). When this happens the personality operates on the basis of unresolved conflicts and wounds that are buried at previous developmental levels. This makes it hard for the conscious personality to access the strengths and riches of those previous levels. For example the mental self can be cut off from the riches of physical vitality or emotional responsiveness. In this way wholeness is damaged and the self leads a one-dimensional existence, starved of vitality and strength.

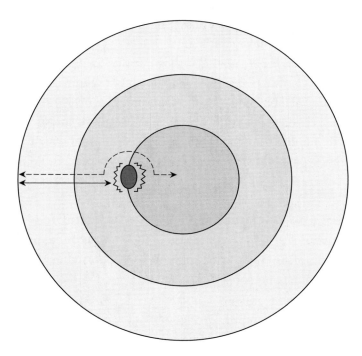

Fig. 5.2 Development and trauma

Traumas at earlier levels of development act like centres of gravity. A wound draws consciousness back to it (just like an itch or burn on your skin) until the wounded part is met, understood and reintegrated. If the wound is at a primal level it also means that one's connection to the source of primal energy is damaged, disturbed or dysfunctional.

Development and Archetype

There is another point that needs to be made here. To say that these stages are simply developmental stages would be overly reductive. Each stage, each world, is also a world in its own right. These worlds have always been there. They are fundamental. They are pre-existent spheres, which humans come to inhabit.

In the past these worlds were imagined as a series of concentric rings. Alchemists and Gnostics imagined the Earth to be surrounded by enclosing worlds, symbolised by concentric rings (see Fig. 5.3). In this view each world is named after an element or a planet. These symbols denote archetypal realities – levels of energy, dimensions of existence – which contain, and exist around, the physicality of the Earth. They said that the soul, in the process of incarnation, journeyed down through these spheres.[35] The soul must then find its way back up through the spheres. In order to become fully conscious it must develop through levels of being.

Because humans have inhabited these worlds for a very long time, they have given these worlds a human face – a human body, human feelings, human thoughts, human society, human culture. So when we grow through the physical, emotional, mental, rule/role worlds and so on, we find a world with a human face to identify with. However, behind each world with a human face stands an archetypal reality, a world of possibilities waiting to be discovered.

Macrocosm and microcosm – the periodic table

The stages or worlds also find expression in the periods of the periodic table. We have seen how the stages of development recognised by developmental psychologists and transpersonal theorists correspond to the seven periods of the periodic table. This worldview is also supported by the imaginative description of levels of reality given by the alchemists.

It is clear that the elements of the periodic table were here long before human beings. All matter is made up of these elements. They are present within the systems and functions of the Earth and all her creatures, including humans.

We can see that these elements are related to different physical and psychological functions. Scientists understand the function of elements such

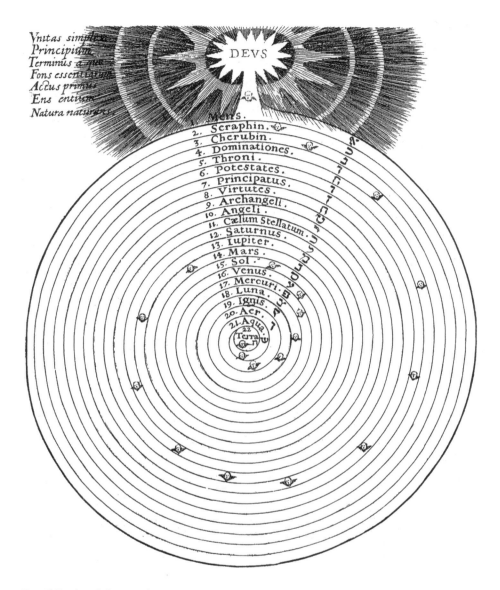

Fig. 5.3 An alchemical vision of consciousness
(from R. Fludd, *Utriusque Cosmi*, Vol. 1, Oppenheim, 1617)

as sodium, iron or iodine. However, many elements (gold for example) have no known function. Even when the physiological function of an element is understood, its psychological function is not understood or recognised.

In homœopathic provings, however, it becomes apparent that every element can derange physiological and/or psychological function. Each element produces a derangement of health characterised by particular alterations in psychological and physical function. This suggests that every element has a role to play in psychological and physical function(s). In other words each element promotes or facilitates a particular function or complex of functions (with physical and psychological dimensions), whether the connection between element and function is currently understood or not.

From our study of the periodic table we can further see that the elements are associated with the sequential unfolding of psychological functions. This sequential unfolding represents the unfolding of consciousness through the developmental stages.

It is as though the elements of each period allow the unfolding of different functions within the human being. For example sodium facilitates water balance. There is also the inner vibrational or psychic dimension of sodium, which facilitates the inner or psychic function of water; namely feelings and feeling relationships.

Another example. Phosphorus is found particularly in the brain and central nervous system. It is through Phosphorus that the "light of reason" becomes possible in the human organism. Phosphorus can thus be thought of as the envoy of the archetypal world of light. Phosphorus anchors the world of light as a human possibility. This possibility/function is encountered by developing consciousness in the developmental stage that we have called the mental/conceptual stage.

Thus the journey of the self is a journey through archetypal worlds or dimensions. This journey is reflected in the elements and periods of the periodic table. Each element facilitates a different function in the human being. Each function has a physical and psychological aspect (water balance and feelings for example). Each of these functions can work healthily or unhealthily. In a proving of an element we see the derangement of the physical and psychological functions connected with that element.

As the Self progresses through the stages of development (and thus through the corresponding periods of the periodic table), dysfunction arises when the consciousness or point of view characteristic of each stage is damaged or wounded. When this happens integration fails to take place as it should.

When there is disintegration in the psyche, bodily dysfunction will follow. We'll take up this last point much more fully later.

Structure of the periodic table

Health depends on access to all the spheres of your make up, not only the current stage of development but also the previous stages contained within it. This idea is mirrored perfectly in the actual structure of the periodic table. With each new period a new shell of electrons is added. Thus all the elements of the first period have one electron shell; all the elements of the second period have two shells; all the elements of the third period have three shells, and so on. With each period the atoms have more weight and depth. Each atom is a functional unit in which all its shells are involved. It is as though the atoms of a particular period contain the previous periods (the previous spheres) within themselves. We, like the atoms, have depth and weight, which must be included in our being.

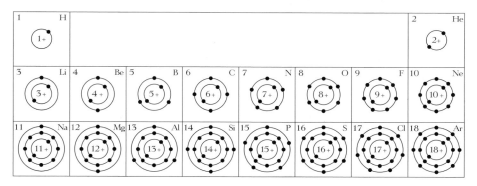

Fig. 5.4 Atoms and electrons: Spheres within spheres. The weight and depth of atoms.

Development and constitution

There is one further point that I must introduce here. The developmental stages constitute a natural progression. To be healthy and integrated each individual must eventually progress through each stage. However, there are stages/worlds in which each individual is more naturally at home. It is as though the soul's preference for a particular sphere of reality is prefigured right from birth (or possibly before birth).

We develop through the stages. At the same time, an individual will have a constitutional affinity for a particular sphere. Thus the analytical Silica individual will have a constitutional affinity, even as an infant, for the mental/conceptual stage of development. There will be a tendency to suffer from the dysfunctions associated with that stage both before and after that stage comes on stream in the developmental sequence. Thus the Silica infant will have a Silica build and Silica likes and dislikes although the developmental stage connected with Silica has not kicked into activity yet.

An important point. Please let's not forget that in homœopathic work we must be guided by the symptoms. What do I mean? In this and the last chapter we have been looking at maps. These maps can help to give depth and context to our understanding of the patient. However it is the symptoms of the patient that must guide to the final choice of remedy. We'll return to this important point more fully in the last chapter.

In the next chapter we'll look at the way in which the body participates in the problems of consciousness.

Chapter 6:
The dynamics of symptom formation

Hahnemann tells us that symptoms – alterations in sensation and function – reveal the distress and "mis-tunement" of the vital force. In this chapter we're going to look at the formation and dynamics of symptoms.

We have seen that as self-consciousness emerges there is, along with potential for consciousness, much potential for damage and imbalance. During the hard-won road to individuality much, for one reason or another, is put aside; potential and creativity that was not nourished; pain that couldn't be dealt with; aspects of ourselves that were denied, neglected or forgotten. In the urge to be oneself and to find one's place in the world, some things are inevitably sacrificed. Aspects of a person can get left behind or wounded. The integrity and harmony of the whole person can be compromised.

Unintegrated aspects of the whole self don't simply disappear, but live an independent life in the unconscious. We have known for a century now that these energies, these aspects of the whole self, can exert a powerful influence on the functioning of the personality in daily life. They cause neurosis and psychosis. And it's not just psychological function that can be disturbed in this way. Homœopathic physician philosophers have always understood the mind and body as a single functioning whole. Although disease is rooted in a person's unconscious feelings, attitudes and beliefs, the symptoms of disease can appear in any part of the whole – mind or body.

What is hidden or repressed in a person is frequently at odds with the conscious personality. Thus a person is often split, in a state of conflict with themselves. Opposing needs and drives pull in opposite directions. Such conflicts are fundamental to human sickness. They lie at the root of human unhappiness and suffering.

Thus all that is in the psyche, but unresolved, unmet or displaced, reveals itself in the presence of symptoms.

Subjective and Objective

We have seen that, broadly speaking, symptoms can be divided into two groups– the subjective and the objective. Subjective symptoms express a condition of consciousness. They take the form of ideas, images, feelings and sensations. In order to understand these symptoms we rely on the descriptive words of the patient. Of course we can also glimpse this subjective world by observing the patient's language, movements, behaviour, and so on.

On the other hand objective symptoms are apparent to the observer. All speech, behaviour, expressions, movements and physical dysfunctions can be classed as objective symptoms.

In order to make a good prescription the homœopath needs to understand the inner and the outer. To understand the outer the homœopath needs to clearly record all that she observes, all that she is told, and all that is revealed through clinical investigation. With patience and discipline this is not hard to do. However, to perceive and record the inner may be more challenging. Will the patient tell us all we need to know? How much of the patient's inner condition is repressed, and therefore inaccessible to consciousness? How skilled is the homœopath in journeying with the patient into the possibly unfamiliar realm of inner experiences, images, feelings and sensations?

Sometimes the patient can speak of their feelings and perceptions without difficulty. At other times we need to help the patient focus on this interior world, especially if the patient is unfamiliar with what goes on inside themselves.

So, if possible, the homœopath needs to perceive the subjective condition of the patient (ideas, images, feelings, sensations) as well as the objective condition (dysfunctions, behaviour, gestures, etc.). However, subjective and objective are really nothing but the inner and outer experience of one phenomenon. Subjective symptoms are our perceptions and inner reactions to something going on in or around us. Objective symptoms are observable dysfunctions. In asthma, for example, tightness in the chest is a subjective symptom (sensation), while laboured breathing is an objective symptom (function).

Images, feelings and sensations – channels to the unconscious

Because unconscious dynamics are so important, the homœopath's senses are drawn to those expressions where the conscious mind has least influence – uncontrived words, images and metaphors; declarations of feeling and attitude that have not been thought about beforehand; dreams and spontaneous associations to dreams; body language; physical sensations and symptoms.

Sensations

Sensations are often evident in acute disease – aching, burning, stitching, and so on. Sensations may be permanently present in chronic disease. In these situations bodily sensations press themselves upon consciousness, demanding to be noticed. All such sensations with their accompanying modalities and localities are carefully recorded by the homœopath.

However, sensations may also be present in a less evident form. The patient may, for example, say that life feels cramped. By inquiring further into the nature of this sensation we can get a clearer idea of underlying sensations which, although not normally conscious, are nevertheless held in the patient's subjective experience. For example when we ask the patient to say what she means by "cramped", she says that her whole being feels constricted or compressed. When she turns her attention inwards she finds that this is her subjective condition (sensation), even though she may not normally be aware of it.

"Is" and "as if"

"Is" and "as if" are equivalent when it comes to the selection of a remedy. What do I mean? For the homœopath it's not of primary importance whether something is actually true, actually happened, or whether it just seems so to the patient. The important point is that the patient reacts as though it were true. Say you've had a fall, feel bruised and don't want to be touched. You need Arnica. On the other hand if you feel bruised from the traumas and difficulties of life and don't want people near you, you may also need Arnica. In the first situation the body actually is bruised. You are bruised and it's obvious. In the second you feel as though you had been hit or injured, even though there has been no physical injury. Furthermore, in this second situation, the injured or bruised sensation will tend to be chronic. Because chronic, it will also tend to be subconscious. Most of the time you will not be aware of the bruised sensation. It is carried deep in the body tissues. These sensations may come to the surface in an acute illness. Failing that, they will only really become apparent when you direct your attention inwards.

Feelings

The patient may be aware of their feelings. In this case they are able to tell us of feelings and emotions that trouble them. However, feelings can be hidden below consciousness causing dysfunction in the body or troubling dreams. Such feelings may rush to the surface during an emotional crisis.

The homœopath needs to make space to allow feelings to come to the surface. The homœopath may need to help the patient to feel and verbalise previously unfelt and unacknowledged feelings.

When the patient is unaware of feelings or sensations (which are nevertheless there below consciousness), he or she can be gently encouraged to go beyond rationalisations and enter the space where they actually feel isolation or anger, or actually experience constriction or floating. This direct experience can in itself be healing for the patient. It also reveals the deep subjective dimension of their sickness. When this subjective data is coupled with symptoms of dysfunction and behavioural changes (the outer symptoms) a more complete picture is revealed.

For example, a woman who was able to access these deeper stratas during the interview found that she felt a deadness, stillness and stiffness (sensations) inside. At this subconscious level she felt unemotional (feeling), in limbo, as though there was no stimulation, no input or output (thought/concept). For this and other reasons (she had been in an abusive relationship) she was given Anacardium orientale. The remedy was of great help to her, and cured her severe headaches.

Images

The unconscious can also reveal itself in images that spontaneously arise (this happens naturally in dreams). This imaginative activity can be an important and revealing part of the homœopathic consultation.

For example one patient described herself as "like a caterpillar that is too big for its skin." She also loved the spring because everything is "bursting out." At this season she would notice plants pushing up through the surface of roads and pavements. These images were charged with dynamic sensation (expansion, bursting, pushing up). They revealed a need for expansion. These descriptions, taken together with specific symptoms and modalities, pointed to the remedy Anhalonium (Lophophora williamsii – the peyote cactus from which mescaline is derived). The remedy had a deeply curative effect.

Images, feelings and sensations are direct channels to the unconscious. They express the condition of vitality (emotion, body and instincts) reflected in the mirror of consciousness. The activity of the vital force arises in consciousness in the form of sensations, feelings and images. Sometimes these are on the surface, accessible to patient and homœopath. Sometimes they are unconscious and need to be uncovered.

It is helpful to remember that when the patient gets to the edge of rationality and thus what can be described by concepts, the perceptions of the patient can jump directly into sensation, feeling or image with very little prompting. It is as though this often ignored and even abused inner world is dying to enter the light of awareness and claim our attention and compassion. The world below consciousness will take any opportunity to reveal itself.

Illusions and beliefs

We must also take into account the illusions and beliefs of the patient. These are often unconscious, deeply rooted, and intractable in the face of reason. They usually relate to the vulnerabilities and experiences of childhood. Because they are unconscious they are often masked and difficult to get at. They surface in a person's dream life or in psychotic states.

For example you might believe you are being victimized. This belief gives rise to a feeling of panic and lack of safety. A person will often repress such thoughts and feelings. Only with inward reflection during the course of the consultation do they become evident. However they can appear in spontaneous remarks like "I always feel that people are after me." Such a person may have dreams of being chased.

Illusions, beliefs, actions and reactions
What is often more evident is someone's reaction to a stressful situation. The basic belief (victimized) is hidden, but reactions to stress (in which the underlying belief is activated) are more visible. Under stress such a person might be easily startled, or have the idea that someone is behind them. They might have an urge to flee, or a sensation of pressure in the chest.

It doesn't matter where these beliefs come from. They may come from childhood experiences. They may come from unresolved ancestral memory patterns. They may even come, as some maintain, from previous incarnations. The point is that they lead you to react as though it were true, as though you were being followed.

Of course if you really are being followed or persecuted, then reacting in such a way is appropriate to the situation. It is a normal reaction. These reactions become pathological when they arise from illusory beliefs. The aim of homœopathic treatment is to free the individual from beliefs, feelings and sensations which are persistent, inappropriate and not related to actual life conditions. This inner healing brings physical healing in its wake.

Practically speaking, if we can see perceptions and actions as two halves of a whole we'll have a better grasp of the case. Often we'll more easily see the action (escape). Then we wonder about the perception/feeling that might give rise to the need to escape. If we hold this in mind we'll be alert for the clues about the feeling or belief behind the action.

Let's recap. On the one hand we have perceptions. These can be in the form of illusions (victimized), images (chased), feelings (abandoned) or sensations (pressure). Out of this arise actions (running). The perception can be general (whole body) or localised (pressure in the chest). If the sensation is pressure in the chest the important thing is pressing.[1] Pressing is occupying consciousness. The fact that it is in the chest shows the domain of "pressing" – inspiration, breathing, air, lungs. However, the perception is in consciousness (consciousness experiences and is identified with chasing or pressing) and is in this sense general, involving the whole person. All of this gives rise to action (see Fig. 6.1 and 6.2).

Thus we have perceptions and actions. Erroneous perceptions lead to erroneous actions. In my understanding this is what Kent meant when he said that disease is a matter of wrong willing (action) which arises from wrong thinking (perception) (see Chapter 7).

Concepts

The descriptions given by the patient will be mixed with the patient's rationalisations and concepts. The rationalisations and concepts about themselves and the world represent the way a person has learnt to cope with inner wounds and life difficulties. We all find reasons and understandings for things. It's important that we go beyond this rational level if we are to understand the underlying dynamics of suffering in the patient.

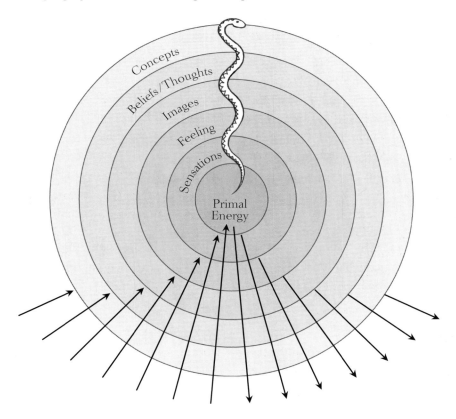

Fig. 6.1 The dynamics of consciousness and symptom formation
The levels form a dynamic whole. Actions arise in response to perceptions.

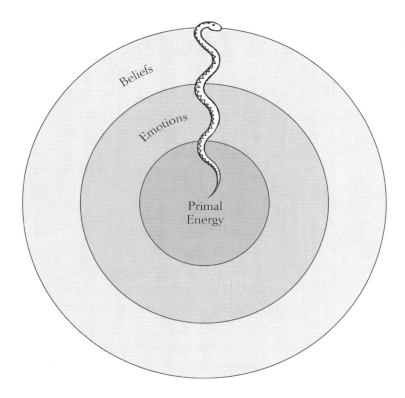

Fig. 6.2 Beliefs/emotions/vitality
Beliefs are energized by emotion, which is rooted in primal energy.

When a person talks about themselves or their problems, they do just that – talk *about* it. The rational mind remains outside the problem, describing it from the outside, like describing a house without actually going inside. Thus the mind with all its rationalisations can be very misleading. The language of the unconscious, of the deeper part of ourselves, is not one of rationality, but of images, feelings and sensations.

Correspondence

What can't be held within the boundaries of one's awareness must eventually appear in the body. This transference from psyche to body occurs through correspondence.

That which is unacknowledged by self-consciousness, reveals itself in the body. There is a dynamic correspondence between above and below. The idea of correspondence is not a new one; in fact, it is a very old idea that has survived into modern times. It was a central idea in the worldview of ancient peoples. Archetypal psychologist and scholar, James Hillman, summarises the history of this way of thinking about the human being in the following passage:

> Already in Egyptian medical ritual there was a relation between specific body organs and specific divine images. In the preparation of the mummy, the lungs were put in an ape-shaped jar, the intestines in a jar with a hawk covering, the stomach with a jackal's head, and the liver in a human-headed jar. Organs were physically located under the 'headings' of divine images or archetypal structures to which they must have been imagined to correspond or belong. Throughout medieval medicine, owing partly to Galen and Islam, different kinds of souls – animal, vegetable, generative, spiritual, blood – were attributed to different regions and systems. In more recent times, Platner (1744 -1818) imagined each major organ to have its own vital force, and Domrich, in the middle of the last century, stressed the relation between specific emotions and specific organs. Toward the close of the last century, Wernicke considered the major organs to have specific symbolic representations. Jung refers to Wernicke's idea and, in his Tavistock lectures, makes several startling diagnostic moves by coupling psychic images and bodily organs. Freud's theory of character traits that are based in different physiologically erogenous zones follows a similar line of thought.[2]

Curiously a giant among these researchers is not mentioned here. We would of course add Hahnemann to the list of those who have explored the nature of the relationship between mind and body. Interestingly enough, the term 'psychosomatic' was coined by Heinroth in 1818, a concept that Hahnemann had been working with for the previous thirty years.

These ideas found a place in the development of homœopathic thought. J.T. Kent writes:

The physical organs correspond to internal man; to the will and understanding. The intellectual faculties consider a proposition presented, weighing it in the light of things learned to determine whether it be false or true, partly false or partly true. The memory holds it while it is examined and considered, and the intellectual faculties digest what is received, separating truth from false, and appropriating the truth and rejecting the false.

The stomach receives food; it and the small intestines digest and assimilate that which is good for the body, and cast off that which is not suitable, that which is indigestible, false. These correspond to the intellectual part of man, doing for the body what the intellectual faculties do for man.

The kidneys perform similar work, separating the false from the true in the blood. The worn out part of the blood is manufactured into urea, urates and is carried off. The kidneys do for the blood what the intellectual faculties do for the truth.[5]

He suggests a correspondence between intellectual and digestive function. A disturbance in the ability to think clearly and process information will be paralleled in the digestive tract by a poor ability to process and assimilate food. I have seen in patients who have difficulty in ordering information on the intellectual level – poor concentration, forgetting words and so on – a corresponding dysfunction (flatulence, indigestion, etc.) in the digestive system that indicates the body is also having difficulty breaking down what it has taken in.

The kidneys separate "the false from the true" in the blood. Kidney function corresponds to the watery world of feelings. Feelings are a kind of instinctive judgement through which we know what is good or bad for us. We often override this knowing with too much rationality.

Kent suggests further that the lungs correspond to intellectual functioning.[4] The word "inspiration" has a double meaning. The body takes in breath. The mind receives ideas. A person can be creatively inspired by "pneuma" or spirit.

Disturbances in all that we associate with the heart – courage, affairs of the heart, love of life – will find expression as pathology of the heart.

Affinities

The homœopathic philosopher physicians of the past understood the notion of correspondence through the idea of affinities. Certain remedies have affinities for certain organs and systems. "The seat of the disease frequently points to the decisive indications [for a homœopathic remedy], for almost every drug acts more definitely upon certain parts of the organism, the whole body seldom being affected equally." [5] Thus Causticum "is a great polycrest remedy, acting upon nerves, motor and sensory, and on muscles, voluntary and involuntary; of bladder, larynx and limbs. Weakness, progressive; loss of muscular strength, causing increasing uncertainty of control over the muscles, finally ending in paralysis; of single organs or parts." [6] Causticum is a potassium salt. Potassium along with sodium is essential for the conduction of nerve impulses. Thus the affinities of Causticum can be seen on the basis of physiological function. However, an understanding of affinities leads to a more comprehensive view. Rajan Sankaran writes, "The Causticum person is very sensitive to any threat to the security of his group and will fight strongly for it ... He can get quite bold and hard externally, though internally he is anxious, nervous, soft. The constant anxiety about his group makes the Causticum person work a lot for others. They need power, control and mobility in order to lead the group and keep it unified; they loose all these – muscular weakness; gradually developing paralysis (very characteristic); stiffness with or without pathologies like rheumatoid and osteoarthritis etc." [7] In other words, the affinity for nervous system and nervous control displayed by the remedy mirrors and gives expression to its psychological preoccupations.

What do these observations suggest? They suggest that a disease process (occurring either as a natural disease or as an artificial disease produced in a proving) finds affinity with particular organs or systems, rendering those organs or systems dysfunctional, because that system of the body has an affinity, an inner connection, with the disturbance in the psyche that lies at the heart of the disease. Thus an issue of power or control, when not met or integrated, may lead to breakdown in the organs of power and control in the body, the muscles and nerves. The primal desires of the heart if repressed or unrecognised can come to expression in heart pathology.

A woman had suffered very severe constipation as a child. She'd always felt unwanted and "pushed to the back". She had been progressing well under treatment for some time and was now having bouts of diarrhoea. When we went into her deeper sensations she became aware of "not knowing when it'll strike". She felt her "sphincters would give, and everything would drop out".

She also felt she'd lost the ability to "hold herself in". However she believed that if "the real me peeps through, people won't want to know me". She felt that she would be unacceptable. She had a sensation of "pressure at the anus, as though something might emerge".

The remedy Aloe socotrina was a turning point and had a remarkable healing effect in her mind and body. In this remedy there is a strong sensation of insecurity in the rectum, as though there is no control over the anal spincter. There are general sensations of fullness and dragging or pressing down, as though something would push out against one's control.

Inwardly they feel that if they relax their real self will come out. They feel then that they would be letting their "shit" out. If that happened people would find them unacceptable or disgusting.

When something is unresolved or unmet in the psyche then a dysfunction of a corresponding or similar nature will appear in the body. This is a kind of dynamic transference whereby an inner disturbance (of consciousness) appears in the outer form of a physical dysfunction.

The practical significance of all this lies in the fact that it helps the homœopath to understand the totality of the sickness and see the way in which apparently unrelated phenomena are part of a single pattern of disturbance.

Projection – the mirror of the world

We must also take into consideration the patient's perceptions of the world about them. This is because our perception of the world is often more a reflection of our own psyche than it is of the world. When we listen to someone's views it often tells us more about the speaker than what they're speaking of.

Much of what we see in the world around us is a projection. In other words, we see events and people through the lens of our own unconscious perceptions. When this happens the world is a reflection of our own internal makeup. We don't see the world as it is.

The law of projection is an important psychological law much discussed by Jung and those who followed him.[8] The law simply says that when something is unconscious, and thus unknown, it is seen as a property of something or somebody in the environment. For example, if I have an unconscious anger that I can't or won't see, then I will see that anger in others. I will blame or criticise others for their anger.

Since most people harbour much that is unconscious, much of what they say about the world around them can be taken as statements about themselves. If a person says, "I hate the way they behave" it is probable that they are saying as much about themselves as about the other person. Thus the homœopath notes statements about other people, objects, animals and so on. These statements are particularly important if they are emphatic or repeated.

In the same way, interests, pastimes, fascinations and obsessions can reflect the preoccupations of the unconscious psyche. A young man who collects knives may well also have a fear of being attacked and stabbed. This fear may be conscious or unconscious.

What we're saying then is that people project aspects of themselves onto surrounding people, objects and events. So, in a sense, statements that someone makes about people, objects and events, especially when emphatic or repeated, can be taken as statements about their own selves. For example if a person refers frequently to another's greed, we can conclude that the speaker has an unrecognised issue around greed. They have a greedy "self" which they ignore or reject. We can take this as part of the patient's picture.

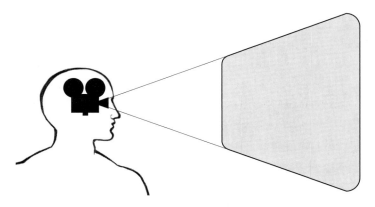

Fig. 6.3 Projection: What's inside is seen outside.

Projection and consciousness

Jung held that projection was an important mechanism in the process of becoming conscious. He said that projection is the mechanism by which that which is unconscious, but needing to be conscious, can become conscious. In other words I first see an unconscious aspect of myself (which nevertheless needs to be more conscious) outside myself. If I am aware that projection is occurring it gives me the opportunity to become more aware of some hitherto hidden dimension of myself. If I reflect on an attitude I have to someone or something (particularly if there are strong emotions involved) it will throw light on my own self. It gives me the opportunity to realise that what I am seeing or feeling says more about myself than the world around me.

Jung saw the taking back of projections as one of the greatest challenges of psychological growth and emancipation.

Polarity and Compensation

Homeostasis is a governing function of all living organisms. Any organism has to maintain equilibrium between opposing forces. For example plants and animals have to maintain integrated functioning within the fluctuating conditions of heat and cold, moisture and dryness, and so on. In other words they have to maintain their stability in an environment of opposing tendencies.

The dynamics of balance and compensation are also fundamental to human life. These dynamics are active in the body and in the mind. They underlie functioning of mind and body. The dynamic level was called by Hahnemann the vital force or "dynamis." [9] The dynamis attempts to maintain rhythmic harmony.

We have seen how, during human development, the rhythmic fluctuation of body and feelings gives way to a choosing self-consciousness. Self-consciousness learns to make judgements between good and bad. We thus find ourselves in a world of opposites. These opposites are often in conflict. Some things are good and some things are bad. We learn to accept the good (what we believe to be good) and keep out the bad (what we believe to be bad). Of course this means that the bad gets worse (more demanding, more offensive, etc.), so the good must become better and stronger in equal proportion.

Polarity strengthens polarity until something breaks. Something breaks down – either psychological well-being or physical health.

Illness arises out of unresolved conflict. Conflict between different parts of ourselves, or conflict between thought and feelings, or between what we "ought" to do and what we desire to do, or between our own feelings and desires and cultural limitations and prohibitions, or between what we want and the physical facts of the world.

Opposites and modalities

It's important to understand the action and relationship of opposites in a case. This understanding has practical applications. For example, sensations and modalities will be equal and opposite to each other.[10] If you feel cold, then heat (the opposite) will ameliorate. More cold makes you feel worse. A person who feels constricted or under pressure will feel better for release or freedom (opposite to constricted, etc.). Homœopathic remedy pictures are full of such examples. Take the snakes. They have a feeling of a lump in the throat (sensation). The response to this is to loosen the clothing around the neck. The greater the sense of internal pressure, the greater the need to loosen the collar. Although tight and loose are opposites, the modality, better from loosening, relieves tightness by allowing expansion. Here the modality works in the same direction as the sensation, rather than against it.

Fig. 6.4 Modalities of aggravation and amelioration need to be equal to the power of the sensation. A modality can be equal in the opposite direction or equal in the same direction.

Another application of the understanding of opposites is in the analysis of a person's general state of being. For example, a boy feels dictated to. He is very sensitive to being bossed around, told what to do. He reacts with obstinacy and resistance. This sensitivity to being dictated to suggests he also has the capacity to be the dictator. He does in fact turn out to be rather bossy and domineering. The issue is dictatorship. The expression can either be sensitivity to it (sensation) or the capacity to do it (action). In casework we would see more of one polarity than the other (sensation of being dictated to, or dictating). However, the other polarity would be there in the background and, given time, would become apparent. Thus, if we are attentive, we will discern an unconscious dominator in the one who is dominated. Sooner or later the dominator will surface. By the same token, one who is dictatorial must also feel dictated to.

All of this becomes important in the selection of rubrics. Thus we find Ferrum metallicum in the rubric "dictatorial", as well as "contradict, disposition to." We naturally want to contradict the one who tries to dominate us. Ferrum has the idea of domination (dictatorial) as well as fighting against perceived domination (contradict, disposition to). So whichever polarity is being displayed, the opposite will be there in the background.

This understanding has technical uses. For example if we find someone is sensitive to being dictated to, but can find no suitable rubric for that sensation, it can sometimes help to go to the rubric that expresses the opposite. Thus it may help to look at a rubric such as "dictatorial." Here we're working on the premise, arising out of our understanding of the action of opposites, that the dictator is sensitive to dictatorship and vice versa. Thus the rubric dictatorial can be taken to mean, "has an issue around dictatorship, one way or the other." An example of this is found in Mercurius. Mercurius is both the dictator (dictatorial) and the anarchist (the one who is sensitive to being dominated and must overthrow the dictator).

Of course the dynamics of polarity are just as evident on the physical level.

Again we can see this pictured in remedies. For example some of the most prominent injury remedies are from the botanical family Compositae (daisies such as Arnica montana, Bellis perennis, Calendula officinalis). If we look at the family as a whole, including other well-known daisies such as Chamomilla and Cina, we see a marked aversion to or aggravation from touch. Arnica has an aversion to being approached. When you approach someone you enter or touch their psychic space. For someone who has been traumatised or injured this can be sensed as potentially threatening or injurious. What these remedies show us is that the experience or sensation of being physically injured or traumatised produces, according to the laws of polarity, an equal and opposite sensitivity or aversion to touch. In a remedy like Chamomilla the perceived threat to safety is so great that the equal and opposite reaction is a need to strike out.

Symptoms as disturbance of natural rhythm

Our bodies may be understood, and felt, as embodiments of rhythm and cycle with their evolutionary roots in the fluctuating life of the natural world. We are biologically rooted in the cycles and seasons of earthly life. In this sense we are embodiments of the world. We are the world internalised.

The emergence of self-consciousness disturbs natural rhythm. Self-consciousness functions through discrimination and polarity. This creates a polarised world of good and bad, light and dark, and so on. This polarity can then disrupt the rhythms of the natural self. Many of the symptoms in the repertory, particularly those of aggravation and amelioration, relate to disturbance of rhythm and function.

When we consider the rhythm and cycles of the body we notice modalities to do with sleep and waking, or to do with the motion or rest of the body. There are also symptoms to do with the effects of eating and drinking. There are the effects of discharges (stool, pus, blood, sweat, menses), suppressed discharges, and from there, different types of discharge. The effects of sexual activity or the lack of it are also important.

When we consider the rhythms and cycles of nature we think of symptoms relating to times of day, light and dark, of season and lunar cycle; also the effects of heat and cold, dryness and dampness, of climate, of geography and atmospheric changes.

Some symptoms are to do with both rhythm of body and world. Sleep and waking for example are rhythms of the body that are tied into the ancient rhythm of day and night. Changes in the rhythmic function of eating, digestion and defecation are alterations of an internal rhythm that is connected to what we take in from the outside.

In disease the healthy rhythms of digestion, breathing, circulation, sexual activity, sleeping and so on become disturbed. Natural rhythm is overturned by polarity. For example sleep can become dysfunctional. There is too much or too little sleep. There is excessive tiredness or excessive wakefulness. There is polarity and imbalance rather than ordered rhythm.

We can see then that the polarities of self-consciousness upset the course of nature both within us and around us. However, and this is one of life's great paradoxes, without this polarising self-consciousness we would not be able to awaken from the sleep of nature.

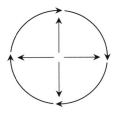

Fig. 6.5 Rhythm and polarity

The economy of health

Control is important to human beings. In order to ensure our own survival and well-being we like to control things in us and around us. Control and judgement go hand in hand. We like to exercise control to keep the good and get rid of the bad.

When it comes to our own selves this means we try to control what comes in and what goes out. For infants and children this control is very important.

The infant or child needs to feel they have control of what enters their physical or psychic space. An obvious way in which an infant can exercise this control is by deciding what food should or shouldn't enter the body.

If, during early life, these physical or psychic boundaries are not established or are in some way violated, the consequences for healthy development can be far reaching.

As well as learning to control what gets in, we learn to try and control what gets out. We learn to hide our true thoughts and feelings. However, what comes in must be balanced by what gets out. If, for example, I eat but don't defecate, I will soon be in trouble. If I experience a grief (input) but don't allow myself to cry (output), well-being will be disturbed. In these instances the basic law of exchange is unbalanced.

The organism is subject to a law of exchange. Incomings and outgoings must be balanced. We receive psychic and physical input. Food must be broken down and assimilated. What is needed is kept and integrated. What isn't needed is discharged. The same can be said for experiences. The impact of a grief must be assimilated. Experiences must be assimilated and emotions discharged. This is a simple law of life. Self-consciousness with its judging and controlling capacities can disturb this economy of incomings and outgoings.[11]

Discharge

There are many levels and types of discharge.

All that is attempting to find form within us must find some sort of expression. To find expression it must be externalised or discharged. Discharges occur in different ways and on different levels. When tension builds up in the emotional system, a discharge of emotion will relieve the tension, like a thunderstorm relieving atmospheric tension. Sexual tension requires a sexual discharge. Creative tension requires a creative discharge – words, song, dance, painting.

Tension and release are the two poles of dynamic function in sentient systems.[12] When there is tension in a psychic or biological system and the necessary discharges are in some way inhibited or thwarted, static energy builds up in that system. Energy that can't flow or find an outlet becomes toxic. It can poison the system. This is true of physical and psychic systems.

Life energy that can't flow creates a number of problems. It can be like a stagnant pool where disease breeds. Or it may, in a different mode of activity, burst out in unpredictable, uncontrollable and inappropriate ways. Thus there may be outbursts of passion or unbridled indulgence. In the body, unintegrated life energies may "burst out" in tumour formation.

The body also needs to discharge the waste products of metabolism. When systems of elimination – bowels, kidneys, skin, mucous membranes – become dysfunctional, toxins build up in the system. The body thus becomes burdened with its own wastes and the necessity of discharge becomes more imperative.

It is interesting that one of the oldest symbols of the life force is the serpent. It represents the rhythmic movement of life energy. But the snake, through its venom, can also destroy living tissue. The snake is thus a fitting symbol of life energy. Life energy is both creative and destructive. Which way it goes depends on the relationship you have with it.

Chapter 7

Individual and Collective

Up to now you might have assumed that all that has been said concerning development and sickness can be put down to problems that originate in the development of the individual. You might have the idea that the individual enters the world as a more or less clean slate, and that problems arise only as a result of the circumstances encountered in this world. This would be a limited perception.

We come into the world unformed and full of raw energy and potential. In this sense we come in to make a fresh start with opportunity before us. But this is not the same as saying that we come in as an empty vessel. When the soul chooses its destiny it chooses to be woven into a larger fabric already woven by ancestors. This isn't only a genetic weave; it's also a weave of thoughts, feelings and desires. What has been developed or undeveloped, thought or not thought, felt and unfelt, done and not done, becomes the material, woven by ancestors, that the soul chooses as the raw material for living.

Miasms

Hahnemann recognised that the individual carries inherited tendencies to sickness. He called these collective foundations of sickness, miasms. This word derives from the Greek word, miasma, meaning a taint, stain or pollution. We now know through the study of genetics that many human characteristics and disease tendencies can be passed on through genetic inheritance. However genetics, like much of science, reduces things to a physical causation. Alter the genes and you alter disease. Miasmatic theory, on the other hand, deals with fundamental patterns that pervade the psychological, cultural and spiritual life of human beings, as well as their genetic makeup.

Let's look in brief at the development of miasmatic theory.

Hahnemann

Hahnemann tells us that in the early days of his practice, despite the discovery and the application of homœopathic principles, many of his patients failed to gain lasting improvement. Although, in many cases, he was able to ameliorate the symptoms, he was unable to bring lasting recovery. He set out to discover why this was, and, he tells us, spared himself no labour until he felt he had found an answer.[1] The answer was his miasmatic theory.

He discovered that behind all chronic disease manifestations lay three basic conditions – psora, sycosis or syphilis. Each one has a characteristic acute contagious manifestation: psora, an itching skin eruption (taking the form in his day of scabies);[2] sycosis, a urethral discharge accompanied by genital figwarts;[3] syphilis, a genital chancre. Through painstaking research of all his cases he uncovered a history (in each individual case) of the suppression of at least one of these acute manifestations. All chronic disease, he maintained, could be traced to the suppression of one or more of these primary acute diseases.

For him these chronic diseases were far more than simple disease complexes. They were fundamental disease patterns that underlay the great variety of apparently separate chronic diseases. These three are like three roots from which arise the great variety of chronic diseases that derange the functions and structures of body and mind.

The most fundamental of the three chronic diseases was the itch disease. When the itching eruption was suppressed it awoke a more extensive internal disease. He believed that the suppression of this acute disease (the itching eruption) awoke an "unknown primitive malady."[4] This malady was, he claimed, the mother of all disease. It was a primal and ancient disease that was awoken from its slumber due to suppression of its primary acute manifestation, the itching skin eruption (scabies in Hahnemann's day, leprosy in about 1500 BC).[5] Even the other basic chronic disease patterns, sycosis and syphilis, could only grow in the soil of psora.

So what have we got here? Let's summarise. Three acute diseases (itching eruption, urethral discharge, genital chancre). These acute diseases are acute contagions that only occur on the basis of a deeper susceptibility in the human being. This susceptibility is due to the three underlying, but slumbering (latent), disease patterns (psora, sycosis, syphilis). Once such an acute contagion appears, so long as it is left alone, the interior health of the individual remains relatively OK. Suppress these acute manifestations and you awaken the fundamental chronic disease patterns. In other words you deny the acute manifestation and thus drive the disease inwards. (Kent later modified Hahnemann's theory of suppression by saying that there was often no evidence of these contagions in a person's history. Rather that the contagions had probably occurred somewhere in the ancestral history. What we receive are the chronic tendencies, which have been awakened by the original suppressions.) These chronic disease patterns then manifest in the great variety of psychological and physical sufferings known to medicine as separate chronic diseases. Behind the great variety of chronic diseases stand the three fundamental chronic disease patterns, psora, sycosis and syphilis. These fundamental patterns are passed on from generation to generation, altering their appearance under the differing circumstances of time and place, *but not altering their fundamental nature.* And at the root of all stands psora.

Psora, this "vast original malady", was called by Hahnemann the "internal itch disease." [6] So what might this "vast original malady", the "internal itch disease", actually be? In previous chapters we have discussed the effect of the emergence of human self-consciousness. We saw how the primary wholeness of nature (including man's nature) is undone by the emergence of self-consciousness (on its way to transpersonal consciousness and conscious wholeness). Thus we lose the guiding thread of life and, as a result of our choosing identity, disrupt nature in and around us. In Chapter 12 I will suggest, in keeping with this hypothesis, that the vast original malady is nothing less that the world-shattering effects of the emergence of human self-consciousness on the evolutionary scene. In terms of human history you can't get much more ancient or primal than that.

The emergence of self-consciousness disrupts the whole. Through self-consciousness we become self-aware, and in becoming self-aware we become aware of our separateness and vulnerability. This produces a primary sense of unease or "dis-ease", a primary unrest or "itch" in the soul. In Chapter 12 we will see how the itch on the skin is at once a symptom of this inner "dis-ease", and a sign of emerging self-consciousness. However, for now we'll stick to this brief history of miasmatic theory with only a minimum of interpretation.

Kent

The nineteenth century physician philosopher, J.T. Kent, gave his own slant to the theory. Psora (the basis of all other disease, including syphilis and sycosis) was, he believed, a primary spiritual sickness. Kent was steeped in the teaching of the spiritual philosopher Emanuel Swedenborg, and saw in the miasmatic theory something akin to the biblical notion of original sin.[7] If we can extract his teachings from their nineteenth century setting, then we come up with something consistent, not only with the teachings of Hahnemann, but with what was suggested earlier in this book.

Kent wraps it up in rather hell and brimstone language:

> As long as man continued to think that which was true and held that which was good to the neighbour, that which was uprightness and justice, so long man remained on the earth free from the susceptibility to disease, because that was the state in which he was created. So long as he remained in that state and preserved his integrity he was not susceptible to disease and he gave forth no aura that could cause contagion; but when man began to will the things that were the outcome of his false thinking then he entered a state that was the perfect correspondence of his interior. As are the will and understanding, so will be the external of man.[8]

In other words, so long as self-consciousness had not emerged to break the charm of nature, things were OK – unconscious, but OK. With the advent of self-consciousness man begins to think and act on the basis of a different criteria than the unconscious rhythm of nature. Thus, in Kent's words, wrong thinking (i.e. the thinking of differentiated self-consciousness which perceives itself as separate from nature), leads to wrong willing, which leads to wrong acting. Put at its most simple, the thinking which arises from a self-consciousness no longer instinctively in tune with the natural way of things, leads to activity which is out of tune with wholeness, which eventually leads to all the dysfunctions that we have come to know as disease.

Ortega

Another important player in this history of miasmatic theory is Proceso Sanchez Ortega, known for his book, *Notes on the Miasms*.

Hahnemann had already stated that all disease symptoms ultimately spring from psora. In his book *The Chronic Diseases*, he devotes many pages to an attempt to list and classify the myriad and diverse chronic symptoms of mind and body that arise as a manifestation of psora. This is an enormous undertaking and presents a problem. When it comes to the miasms as a method of classification of types of disease (psora, sycosis and syphilis) and the remedies that correspond to those grand disease patterns, this amount of data is obviously unmanageable. What's needed instead of lengthy lists of symptoms as characteristic of each miasm, which have to be memorised by the practitioner if they are to employ the theory in clinical practice, is an understanding of the essential pattern running through the group of symptoms characteristic of each miasm. Ortega has given us just such an understanding.

He says, look, if you take each grand group of symptoms as a whole, what do you see? You see three fundamental disease patterns manifesting in both mind and body. Psora is characterised by deficiency, lack and hypofunction. Sycosis is characterised by excess, exuberance and hyperfunction. Syphilis is characterised by perversion, destruction, degeneration and aggression.[9] In short, too little, too much, and destruction. We'll return to the significance of this shortly.

Sankaran

Rajan Sankaran has made further important contributions. According to him the keynote of psora is anxiety about one's ability to cope with life. This gives rise to a struggle to succeed, although the psoric is hopeful that he will succeed. Sankaran says of the sycotic miasm; "It is a feeling of a fixed, irremediable weakness within oneself. With this admission, there is an attempt to cope with it by covering it up, and hiding it from others by egotism, secrecy and compulsive acts." [10] He describes the syphilitic miasm like this; "The delusion of syphilitic remedies is that they are faced with a situation that is beyond salvage, leading to complete hopelessness and despair." [11] The concomitants to this mindset are violence and destruction.

Sankaran, like others before him, has added other miasms to the basic three. If we take the basic three as a sequence – psora, sycosis, syphilis – he has added further miasms that lie at intervals between the main three. They represent points that lie before psora, or between psora and sycosis, or between sycosis and syphilis. This extended model, which we'll return to later in the chapter, doesn't alter the idea of the basic three. It takes the basic three and breaks them down into further subdivisions. Instead of cutting the cake into three parts, Sankaran cuts it into ten parts. Sankaran's sequence of miasms is acute, typhoid, psora, malaria, ringworm, sycosis, cancer, tubercular, leprosy and syphilis. [12]

Let's summarise the characteristics of the basic three before continuing.

Summary of the three miasms

Psoric

There is withdrawal, timidity and anxiety in the face of life. There is a fundamental fear that is based on a primal feeling of separation and loss. There is a sense of lack and of loss with accompanying fear of life and the future. In compensation to this there is struggle to succeed. Physical deficiency shows itself as lack of vitality, chilliness, dryness, hypofunction of organs and systems. The outward expression of psora is the itching skin eruption. This outer itch arises from a more fundamental inner sense of anxiety and disquiet (see Chapter 12).

Sycotic

According to Sankaran the sycotic believes they have an inner weakness that cannot be altered. All you can do is hide it. One covers it up with fixed attitudes and rigid behaviour. However, repressed life becomes "hideous"; something we want to hide and are ashamed of. This makes a person frightened and mistrustful of their own life force. We fear that what we let out, our sexuality, our spontaneity, our creativity, will not be normal. This need to control the spontaneity and expression of the life force leads to rigidity of the personality and a proneness to guilt. Thus a tendency to fixation in thought and attitude, coupled with a feeling of shame and a need to keep control of what are felt to be unacceptable characteristics are the hallmarks of the sycotic personality. The opposite polarity can be unbridled indulgence and greed, repressed vitality having broken free of all controls. Physically there is hyperfunction – copious catarrhal discharges from any mucous surface, tumour and wart formation.

Syphilitic

The characteristic of the syphilitic miasm is destruction. Psychologically there is violence, rage and hatred. There is a feeling that others are trying to destroy you. Or there is a desire to destroy others and even to destroy oneself. There is despair and hopelessness. Physically there is ulceration and necrosis.

Why should the syphilitic pattern establish itself? In the stage of endings disintegration is natural. However if a person attempts to hold on to and maintain something that is ending (that is to say, dying), they can become paranoid and defensive. They become stuck in the place of death and destruction.

Sequence of the miasms

In this summary of the miasms we can start to discern a sequence. Psoric feelings of failure and struggle to succeed arise naturally at the start of something new, at the start of a new phase of life or experience. Sycosis is more to do with getting established and the accompanying need to hide or deny parts of oneself that don't fit with established identity. Syphilis points more to endings, and to what happens when natural disintegration is resisted.

Thus this view of the miasms begins to look like a simple pattern of beginning, middle and end. For a human life this means birth, life (and desire for life) and death.

This beginning, middle and end pattern applies to all that is born, lives and dies – to things, feelings, ideas, people, civilisations, planets. However, staying with the cycle of a human life, the miasms can be further summarised like this:

Psora

Birth, loss of union. Grief, sense of loss, desire to go back. Anxiety about capacity to go forward, to succeed. Withdrawal, or struggle to succeed. Hypofunction.

Sycosis

Life. Getting established; repression and control of everything that doesn't seem to fit the status quo. Thus hiding and cover up of unruly naturalness and desire (love, life). Or conversely, unbridled life, too much life, too much love (hyperfunction); i.e. the breakout of suppressed life, love and desire.

Syphilis

Death – the end of a cycle; the need for death, but resisting death; therefore courting death and destruction; violence, hatred and destructive processes. (Death also leads to reunion in the sense that death is a going beyond form; return to the formless.)

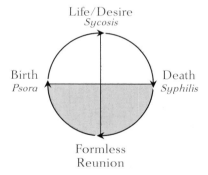

Fig. 7.1 The miasm cycle and the circle of life

We must be careful not to see all this as merely pathological. We have seen that the cycles of birth, life and death pervade all aspects of our life. No birth means no desire, means no life. Creation, and all that is created, displays all its magnificence in its desire for life and yearning for the beloved. Rose petals open in a gesture of the most sensuous desire for the touch of raindrops and the warmth of sun. All that is created burns with desire and weeps from the exquisite pleasure and pain of the longing to go home to the One that always was, is and always will be. And death is the end of struggle and longing as we are swept up again in the loving arms of unfathomable love and mystery.

But all this birth, living and dying has become a source of distress and suffering for us humans on the slow, magnificent and awful, loving and terrible road home. Because we can no longer fall on our knees in the great initiatory rites of birth, love and death, the presence of birth, love and death have become diseases. The Fates have become diseases.

Miasms, stages of development and the periodic table

The pathology of the miasms seems to relate to birth and beginnings, life and desire, and death and endings. All of life is in the process of being born, of living and dying. There are cycles of birth, life and death going on in us and around on every scale and level of existence from microcosm to macrocosm. In our own lives things are living and dying constantly – the cells of our bodies, our feelings, our ideas, our beliefs, our possessions. In fact all that we identify with is continually being born, living and dying.

I'd like now to turn our attention again to the emergence of self-consciousness. We saw that when it comes to the unfolding of a human life, the stages of development in human self-consciousness are particularly important. Each of these stages is itself a cycle with a beginning, a middle and an end. Each stage engages emerging self-consciousness in a new round of birth, life and death.

Miasms and stages of development

We have seen that each stage in the development of consciousness is characterised by three phases. In phase one it is necessary to grow into the new stage of development. The challenge must be met. There is struggle to adapt, to assimilate and to succeed. There is also a fear of failure and a desire to turn back, to shrink away from the new stage of individuation. This is the psoric phase.

In phase two, consciousness establishes itself in the new stage. This stage now becomes the focus of consciousness. It is the reality that consciousness identifies with. For example, in the second (middle) phase of the mental/conceptual stage the self has met the challenges of growing into the mental/conceptual world of image, thought and concept and is now particularly identified with thoughts, concepts and thus with self-image. In this phase how one sees oneself (and how one is seen by others) becomes the pervasive and all-important reality. This is the sycotic phase of the mental/conceptual stage.

The third phase is one in which the self dis-identifies with the current stage of development, which in the natural order of things involves the ending of that stage of development and the necessity for birth into the next stage. One has to let go, rather than hold onto something that is disintegrating. This is the syphilitic phase.

Miasms and the periodic table

Each series of the periodic table also has an initial phase, a middle phase and a phase of decline (these phases are subdivided into eighteen phases which represent eighteen points on the wave of ascent, peak and descent).

Each period of the periodic table has a phase of birth/struggle, a phase of establishment/maintenance, and a phase of decline/disintegration. Thus the three phases of each developmental stage of consciousness correspond more or less with the beginning, middle and end of each series of the periodic table (see Fig. 7.2 and 7.3).

Scholten has shown that the remedies at the left-hand end of the table correspond to the difficulties of beginnings and getting started (in any particular series). The remedies in the centre represent the peak of the development of that series, and the remedies towards the right-hand end represent the gradual decline and ending of the developmental wave.

What about the miasms? We have established that the miasms also belong to beginning, middle and ending. Psora is characterised by the doubt and struggle that is encountered at the beginning of any undertaking. Sycosis is characterised by the covering up of what is felt to be unacceptable (often repressed instincts and life drives). This is felt as necessary to survival or acceptance in the phase of establishment. Syphilis is characterised by decay, destruction and despair; the stance of the syphilitic is the stance of the self faced with the inevitability of death and ending.

If all this is so then remedies that are known particularly as psoric should be found more in the left side of the periodic table (beginnings, birth),

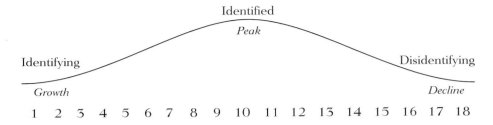

Fig. 7.2 The periodic wave (after Scholten, 1996, p. 29)
Seen as three phases and eighteen stages.

remedies that are sycotic should be found more in the middle of the table (establishment, cover up) and remedies that are syphilitic (ending, destruction) should be found more towards the right hand end of the table. Can we see any correspondence here?

If we take the mineral remedies that are known as syphilitic or as having a strong syphilitic component, they do indeed mostly belong to the right hand end of the table. Among the most notable syphilitic remedies are Nitric acid, Fluoric acid, Phosphorus, Arsenicum (especially Arsenicum iodatum), Aurum metallicum (also Aurum muriaticum) and Mercurius. We can see that they're all in the right hand half of the chart.

On the other hand some of the most prominent psoric remedies are at the left-hand end of the chart; Natrum muriaticum, Natrum carbonicum, Alumina, Kali carbonicum, Calcarea carbonica, Baryta carbonica.

This leaves the sycotic remedies. Silica (vertical column ten) is psoric/sycotic.[14] It has the withdrawal of psora as well as fixation and cover up of sycosis. Palladium is also a sycotic remedy.[15]

What we can say then is that there seems to be a predominance of psora at the left-hand end of the periodic table, a predominance of sycosis in the middle, and a predominance of syphilis at the right-hand end.

The vertical axis
There is also a vertical movement, which involves a descent through the periods of the table that correspond to the early stages, the middle stages and the later stages of the development of self-consciousness. This might be seen as a movement from psora as the beginning of self-consciousness, to sycosis as

144

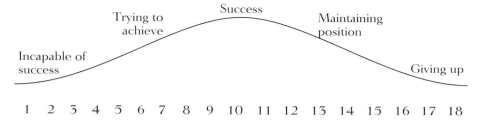

Fig. 7.3 The periodic wave

Another way of looking at the wave. Sankaran gives five phases.[13]

the establishment of self-consciousness, and thence to syphilis as the disintegration of self-consciousness.

It is certainly true that carbon gives any carbonate remedy a psoric character (like Calcarea carbonica for example). Silica belongs to the mental/conceptual stage of development in which, along with self-image, repression and self-denial become more definite possibilities. Silica belongs to the third period and has a strong sycotic component.

There is no doubt that the heavy metals are more strongly syphilitic. The themes of death and destruction are stronger here.

The ten miasms

Any life cycle has a beginning, middle and end. We have seen that these three phases correspond to psora, sycosis and syphilis. In the periodic table this sequence of three is subdivided into eighteen phases.

Sankaran has extended the idea of the basic three miasms. He has put miasms in-between the basic three. This is because, in his view, there are more than three basic categories of perception and reaction seen in individuals. So for him the basic three-miasm model becomes a ten-miasm model. From the perspective of the cycle model suggested in this chapter we can now talk of ten phases rather than three. The ten phases represent a further way of subdividing the life cycle of beginning, middle and end (just as the periodic table subdivides the basic cycle into eighteen phases).

Everything is cyclic. Everything is born, grows and dies. The number of points we put on the cycle (like the marks on a clock face) is a matter of what works in practice. In the case of the periodic table this number is eighteen, because it reflects the structure of the periodic table. Sankaran has arrived at ten miasms on the basis of the observation that people show ten basic modes of perception and reaction in life situations. He has hinted at the cyclic nature of this model by designating an age to each miasm.

If we view each miasm as a stage of a cycle then each miasm lies somewhere in the cycle between beginning and end. Each individual has a propensity to experience difficulty or conflict at one point of the cycle or another. Regardless of the situation (job, relationship, a project, etc.) each individual has a tendency to cope as though they were at the beginning (or in early phases), or as though something were accepted and established, or as though something were declining. Problems come at the beginning, middle or end, or at one point or another in-between. Each phase or miasm thus has its characteristic posture.

I'll introduce Sankaran's ten miasms now, and come back to them again in Chapter 13.[16]

The first miasm is the *acute*. There is a feeling of sudden danger or threat – the kind of feeling you might get when faced with a sudden threat to your life, as for example in an earthquake. The reaction is panic or escape. Aconite belongs to the acute miasm.

The second, the *typhoid* miasm, lies between the acute and psora. The feeling is one of a sudden (acute) loss of a position of comfort, with a need for an intense short effort (psora) to resolve the situation. Bryonia belongs to the typhoid miasm.

The *psoric* feels he needs to struggle to reach his goal; a goal that he is nevertheless hopeful of achieving.

The *malaria* miasm falls between the acute and the sycotic. They feel limited, persecuted and unfortunate. Their acceptance of the situation (sycotic) is punctuated by intermittent attacks of anger or rage (acute). Natrum muriaticum and China are good examples of remedies that belong to this miasm.

In the *ringworm* miasm one alternates between struggle (psora) and resignation (sycosis).

The *sycotic* accepts the situation and tries to cover up what he sees as being wrong with him. Thuja and Pulsatilla are typical remedies.

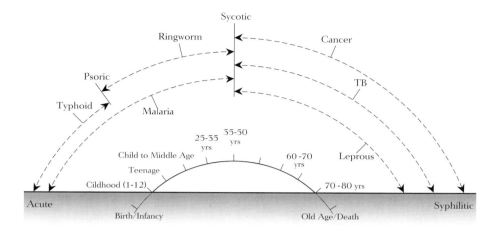

Fig. 7.4 The cycle of the miasms (after Sankaran, 2002, Vol. 1., pp 53 and 66-69)
Sankaran gives a suggested typical age for each miasm. This doesn't mean that at a particular age you are in the equivalent miasm. However it does suggest that the miasm represents the stance and difficulties typical for a certain age. For example the acute miasm is normal in infancy. The sycotic stance is normal for middle years. A stance becomes pathological (i.e. miasmatic) when it is habitual. One can be predisposed, through inheritance, to any habitual (miasmatic) pattern, at any age.

The *cancer* miasm lies between sycosis and syphilis. These people feel faced with a superhuman task. Therefore control and perfectionism are hallmarks of the cancer miasm. They sense that things are disintegrating. They try to control the inevitability of disintegration with control (particularly self-control) and perfectionism. Carcinosin and Arsenicum album are typical of the cancer miasm.

The *tubercular* miasm also lies between sycosis and syphilis. The feeling is of being caught or suffocated, with a desperate need for change. Tuberculinum and Phosphorus are two typical remedies.

The *leprosy* miasm is going towards syphilis. One feels shunned, despised and isolated. Aloe socotrina belongs to this miasm (see Chapter 6).

The *syphilitic* is characterised by despair and destruction. Mercurius is typical.

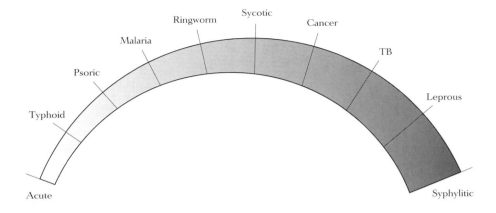

Fig. 7.5 The depth and pace of the miasms.[17]

As the personality matures it deepens. Likewise the miasms take a progressively deeper hold. In the spectrum from acute to syphilitic the consciousness of suffering becomes progressively deeper and more chronic.

In summary

We live in a world that surrounds us, above, below and to the sides, with birth, life and death. We are constantly living out our own dramas of birth, life and death. We carry ancestral memories of birth, love and death; ancestral memories of births, desires and deaths lived through, ignored, unrecognised, messed up, not honoured, and so on. This is our miasmatic inheritance.

We must replay the drama of birth, establishment and death through every stage of our development. We must walk the circle of life many times until we remember that we're here to love the circle of life while knowing that in essence we do not die and are never born.

In healing we need to attend to the old patterns, which we carry in the form of psora, sycosis and syphilis. We need also to remember to attend to all that is being born, all that is living, loving and desiring, and all that is ending, decaying and dying within and around us. When we do this we live our destiny and honour the Fates.

In the next chapter we will look at the way in which the powers of nature are embodied in our constitution.

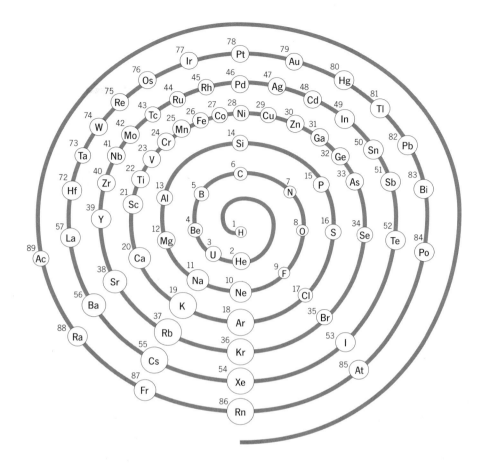

Fig. 7.6 Periodic table as spiral of life

When the periodic table is viewed as a spiral we can see that each element/remedy is simply a stepping-stone (which we might fall off or otherwise fail to negotiate) in the unfolding and awakening of our individual consciousness to the one unbroken reality that gives birth to the dance of the elements and the dream of life.

Chapter 8:

Approaches to constitution (part one): Three levels of being

The word "constitution" refers to the composition or make up of something – the elements that make up the whole. In Chapter 2 we looked at human constitution in terms of the relationship between nature and consciousness. We then considered the way in which human self-consciousness emerges out of the matrix of nature. The relationship between nature and human consciousness has not always been a successful marriage.

Human constitution may also be thought of as having three spheres or levels. This idea is found in many systems and traditions. We think of ourselves as constituted of mind, emotions and body. In the Ayurvedic system there are three fundamental human types – the vata type, the pitta type, and the kapha type. In Hindu philosophy there are three paths to enlightenment – the way of knowledge (head), the way of the heart (heart), and the way of karma or duty (action). Paracelsus said there were three elements in human makeup – mercury (spirit), sulphur (soul) and salt (body).[1]

Rudolph Steiner, the founder of Anthroposophy, also held that the human being has a threefold constitution. He called these three elements of constitution the nervous constitution, the rhythmic constitution and the metabolic constitution. The nervous constitution is centred in the cranial cavity, its organ is the nervous system and it is concerned with thinking and consciousness. The rhythmic constitution is centred in the thoracic cavity. Its organs are the lungs, heart and circulation. It is concerned with feelings, emotion and rhythmic activity. The metabolic constitution is centred in the abdominal cavity. Its organs are the organs of digestion. It is concerned with building and breaking down. It is also, according to Steiner, the seat of the will.[2]

In the nervous constitution lies our choosing nature. In the rhythmic constitution lies our rhythmic and functional nature. In the metabolic constitution lies our capacity to build and maintain a form. Put simply this gives us a threefold view of the human being – consciousness, function and structure.

In the condition of asthma with laboured breathing and a sensation of pressure in the chest (see Chapter 6), pressing is a condition of consciousness (pressing is occupying awareness) and laboured breathing is a disturbance of the respiratory function. This is located in the respiratory structure, the lungs. Consciousness (pressing), function (breathing) and structure (lungs).

Animal, plant, mineral

We can also look at the threefold constitution of the human being in terms of a mineral, plant and animal constitution. Esoteric traditions have recognised that the human being contains within them the mineral, plant and animal kingdoms.[3] In our makeup there is something mineral-like, something plant-like and something animal-like.

These ideas have been taken up by contemporary homœopaths such as Rajan Sankaran and Chaim Rosenthal.[4] They have suggested that differential diagnosis in remedy selection can be aided through an understanding of the general characteristics of remedies from each kingdom.

There are three levels – the mineral, the plant and the animal (they might be called mineral soul, plant soul and animal soul). Each needs to be in the right relationship with each other and with human consciousness. Because these three levels are present in the human being, in disease we will see signs of dysfunction in each level, the mineral, the plant and the animal. However, the focus of the problem will be more on one particular level than the others. One level or another will be particularly stressed, damaged or unintegrated. This points to a remedy from that kingdom – mineral (including liquids, gases, etc.), plant or animal.

Human

The human being is a holon with a mineral nature, a plant nature, an animal nature and a human nature. Evolution on this planet has progressed from the mineral, through plant and animal, to the human. The mineral world is the world of form and is most evident in the structure of the body. The plant world is the world of adaptation, reactivity and procreation. It is most evident in the rhythmic functions of body and feelings, and in processes (physical and psychological) of adaptation and exchange with the environment. The plant world brings the mineral world alive.

In the animal world desire, power and assertion of self come into play. In the animal world the mineral and plant levels are endowed with motion, emotion, desire and self-interest. The animal world is present in human constitution as desire, passion and individual assertion.

The human level represents the integration of the three previous levels. At the human level there is the potential for the three kingdoms to work together as a more integrated and more conscious whole.

Human being	Paracelsus	Steiner	Levels of being	Kingdom
Spirit	Mercury	Nervous	Consciousness	Animal
Soul	Sulphur	Rhythmic	Function	Plant
Body	Salt	Metabolic	Structure	Mineral

Fig. 8.1 The three spheres of human existence – different perspectives compared

Let's summarise the characteristics of each kingdom.

Mineral
The mineral kingdom is structural and fundamental. Keywords are structure, foundation, organisation, systematic. The person needing a mineral remedy is concerned with structure and support. Their structure/support is threatened. This might be the structure of their home, job, family, identity or ideas.

Plant
The plant is a living whole. It is enlivened, dynamic structure. A plant has to maintain form and function as a living whole within fluctuating environmental conditions. It has to be able to adapt. In order to adapt it has to be sensitive to environmental changes (moisture, temperature, light, etc.). Relationship and exchange with the environment are important.

Keywords for the plant kingdom are sensitivity, adaptability, reactivity, vulnerability (the plant cannot alter the environment, it can only adapt). In the person needing a plant remedy there is sensitivity and changeability. Their sensitivity and adaptability are threatened. Therefore they feel vulnerable, easily influenced, easily affected and easily hurt. According to Rajan Sankaran this sensitivity is expressed especially in the form of sensations.[5] The patient's sensations express his or her vital sensitivity and need for adaptation.

Animal

The animal kingdom is concerned with territory, aggression, power and sexuality. Domination and being dominated are important. Territory and mating are important. Protection and nurture of the young are important. In the animal kingdom we see the establishment of individual supremacy over other individuals or in a group. Thus we might say that the assertion of individuality is central to the animal kingdom. Therefore the person needing an animal remedy feels a threat to their consciousness of self. They feel a threat to their sense of individual identity, individual attractiveness or individual power.

Keywords for the animal kingdom are competition, attractiveness, victim/aggressor. There is also conflict between the animal side (desire, sexuality, aggression, etc.) and the human side (reason, self control, etc.).

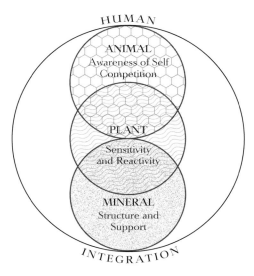

Fig. 8.2 The holarchy of the three kingdoms

In summary then, in the mineral kingdom structure and support are threatened. It is the mineral basis that is threatened or poorly integrated. In the plant kingdom sensitivity and adaptability are threatened. It is the vital level that is compromised. One experiences threat to or difficulty in vital function. This is experienced in the form of painful or uncomfortable sensations. In the animal kingdom it is the individual sense of consciousness, the individual sense of self that is threatened or wounded.

Each of these levels represents a mode of being in the world. Obviously each mode is present in each person. However, one mode of being can stand out more than others. When this is apparent it may help the homœopath in the differential diagnosis between remedies.

There are three modes of existence in the world. Just existing (mineral), reacting and adapting (plant) and self-assertion (animal). These modes are closely related to four primary conditions posited by the philosophers of the ancient world. These are the elements fire, air, water and earth. We'll look at these in the next chapter.

Chapter 9:

Approaches to constitution (part two): Four elements

In this chapter we'll look at the four elements spoken of in classical Greek and other traditional philosophies – earth, water, fire and air.

The ancients believed that everything was composed of these four (sometimes five) elements. We now know of course that the cosmos and everything in it is made of one hundred or so elements, the elements of the periodic table. We also know that these elements themselves are made up of subatomic particles – neutrons, protons and electrons. It is further posited that there are yet more elementary particles such as quarks.

The elements of modern science are in us and around us, and we can often touch, see or smell them (carbon in your fireplace, noxious gases, and so on) but they don't really speak to the imagination in such a fundamental way as the four traditional elements.

Fire, air, water and earth are immediate experiences. We often need specialist knowledge to know about oxygen, copper and arsenic. Even when there is common experience and imagination surrounding an element such as iron, sulphur or gold, the experience of these things is not as everyday, not as immediate, not as total as it is of fire, air, water and earth. We can see and touch the four elements in the world around us. We can also experience heat, cold, dry and wet as immediate subjective experiences. The elements pervade the most basic sense of ourselves and the world. The language of the elements underpins the imagination. We talk about being fired up, all at sea, airy-fairy or down to earth. We also encounter the primal elements in our dreams.

These primal elements belong to the realm of the preverbal, pre-conceptual psyche. In other words they belong to the bedrock of the earliest stages of experience. As we saw in Chapter 4 (and know from the work of Stanislav Grof), the primal experiences of ourselves and the world are elemental. During the birth experience, images of deluge and volcano flood the psyche, as do sensations of compression, release, heat, cold, and so on. The infant psyche experiences a world of elemental sensations.

The elements also relate to the stages of consciousness discussed in previous chapters. Conception is fiery. Intrauterine existence is watery. The development of the physical self belongs mostly to earth. The feeling self belongs to water. The mental/conceptual self belongs to air.

An awareness of the elements also helps us to understand how psychological processes correspond with physical processes. For example, through an awareness of the elements we can understand how unshed tears might be related to oedema or kidney dysfunction.

Awareness of elemental correspondences can also throw light on the relationship between the patient's internal condition and the environment. For example a person who is waterlogged – physically or emotionally – might feel worse in cold wet weather. When inner waterlogging meets oppressive dampness, the patient feels worse.

History

In cultures of the past it was understood that the individual, human culture, the life of nature, and the being of the cosmos were all embedded in one single reality. This reality was understood to be the expression of the cyclic activity of archetypal energies. These powers are operative in the life of nature and cosmos. They also play through all spheres of human activity.

In ancient China, for example, it was understood that two primary principles stood behind the world of cyclic phenomena. These are male and female or yin and yang. Various combinations of yin and yang in turn give rise to further dynamic possibilities.

Thus the philosopher scientists of ancient China were able to create a map of the activity of these primary powers. They used a circular diagram – the universal compass – to depict the relationship of powers. The trigrams

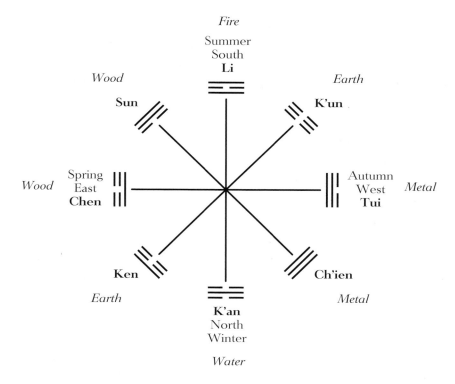

Fig. 9.1 The world compass of trigrams (Later Heaven, or Inner-World Arrangement (after the Richard Wilhelm translation of the I Ching)

(the primary combinations of yin and yang) are arranged in pairs of opposites to correspond with season, compass direction and element. The primary powers are seen not as polarised opposites – this is what they become in the imbalance of human sickness – but as phases of a dynamic and cyclic movement in which conditions are transformed and give way to each other. Summer and winter, for example, are not seen as mutually exclusive opposites, but as phases of a cyclic activity in which one set of conditions is transformed into its own opposite and back again in an unbroken dynamic.

The cyclical movement of primary energies is understood to be operative in all phenomena; in night and day, in the seasons, as well as in human culture and thought. As well as this, different phenomena are seen to be in correspondence. Thus the south, summer and fire are all different expressions of the trigram "Li." They correspond to each other.

This understanding is elaborated in the ancient text of the I Ching, the Chinese Book of Changes, which seeks to reveal the patterns of cyclical dynamic change in nature and human life. Reference to the I Ching can help one to see a particular life situation as part of a larger dynamic pattern. The idea is that this should lead to understanding and appropriate action. In a similar way the homœopath sees a symptom – an apparently isolated health "event" – as an expression of the movement of an underlying dynamic energy, through which all is woven into a single whole.

The four conditions of constitution
In the Western tradition of inquiry the Greek philosopher Empodecles introduced the idea of the four elements in the fifth century BC. This system was also central to Platonic philosophy. These early philosophers understood the four elements as the four fundamental conditions or states of being of which all manifest reality was composed. The elements were understood as archetypal essences present in all phenomena. Similar ideas are to be found in ancient Egypt.

The idea of the four elements was further developed by Hippocrates and Aristotle. They took the basic model and used it to help them understand human constitution in health and disease. This gave rise to the idea of four associated humours (gall, black bile, phlegm and blood), and four associated conditions (wet, dry, hot and cold). The philosopher physicians of the middle ages added the idea of the four temperaments as well as corresponding colours, seasons, tastes, foods, plants and organs.

The idea of the four humours was used and elaborated in medicine right up to the recent past. The idea of the temperaments (sanguine, choleric, melancholic and phlegmatic) is part of our cultural inheritance. These ideas were revitalised by Rudolph Steiner in the early twentieth century. Around the same time Jung established that there are four modes of psychological functioning – intuition, thinking, feeling and sensation.[1] These four functions relate to the four elements.

Mappa Mundi – a map of the inner and outer world

The map presented in this chapter was developed by Misha Norland on the basis of the work of homœopath Joseph Reves. It draws on traditional Chinese and Western philosophy and understanding of the world. Some homœopaths use it to help them understand the inner dynamics of a particular remedy or the inner pattern at work in a person's sickness. (For more on the map, its history and uses, see the work of Misha Norland and Joseph Reves.[2])

Chinese philosophy related elements, seasons and compass points together. This map goes a little further. It relates the elements with human temperament and with various conditions of the mind and body. It helps in seeing psychological disposition, physical type and physical pathology as a single whole.

The Mappa Mundi (map of the world), then, is primarily a map of the relationship of the four elements. To this has been added the four temperaments and their associated qualities – conditions of heat and cold, wet and dry. The corresponding seasons, compass points, times of day and colours are also added. As well as this the axes of spirit (vertical) and matter (horizontal) are shown. Also polarities of opening and closing and of movement and stillness are shown. Psychological qualities and physiological functions are also included.

The map shows the elements as being in us and around us. It shows us that we are made of the stuff of the world. It shows that human constitution is an expression of the constitution of the world. We are made of one and the same stuff. Fire, air, water and earth exist in us and around us. They are present around us in the life of nature. They are present in the functioning of our bodies. They underpin psychological imagery.

We now know, through knowledge of the periodic table, that we are quite literally made of the same stuff as the earth, seas, atmosphere and stars.

However, this map shows us that behind the elements known to science stands a dynamic pattern that is an interplay of forces. It is this interplay of forces (the elements of antiquity) that the sages of East and West sought to picture in their maps.

The map

Looking at Figure 9-2a we see at the cardinal points the correspondence of an element, a psychological function (thinking, feeling, etc.), a compass point, a colour, a taste, a quality (hot, dry, etc.), and a time of day. We also see the axes of spirit and matter. At the mid-cardinal points we see a combination of two qualities (hot and dry, cold and wet, etc.) corresponding with a time of day, a season, a phase of life, as well as a colour. We also see the axis of expansion (opening) and contraction (closing) and the axis of action (dynamic) and stillness (static).

Figure 9-2b shows, at the cardinal points, the correspondence of an element (the heat process, etc.) with psychological qualities and physical systems and functions.

Figure 9-2c shows the correspondence of a temperament with a humour. For example the sanguine temperament, which is hot and wet, corresponds with the blood (hot and wet), and the spring (hot and wet). Each temperament is shown with associated psychological characteristics and physical systems and functions. An associated modality is shown, along with associated images.

Thus the map links human qualities with seasons and times, with colours, tastes, elemental conditions, and with the cycle of a human life from birth to death.

The map can be used to look at cases or remedy pictures. Let's look at some examples of well-known remedy pictures. I've chosen four that all homœopaths will be familiar with. I've put them in pairs that are known for their complementary relationship with each other – Bryonia and Natrum muriaticum, Belladonna and Calcarea carbonica (see Fig. 9.3 to 9.6). These examples will help us to see how the map hangs together, as well as giving an insight into the dynamics of each remedy. It will also throw light on their complementary relationship. These short examples are intended to give an idea of the dynamics that underlie the symptom picture of each remedy. They are not meant as comprehensive pictures. They're thumbnail sketches.

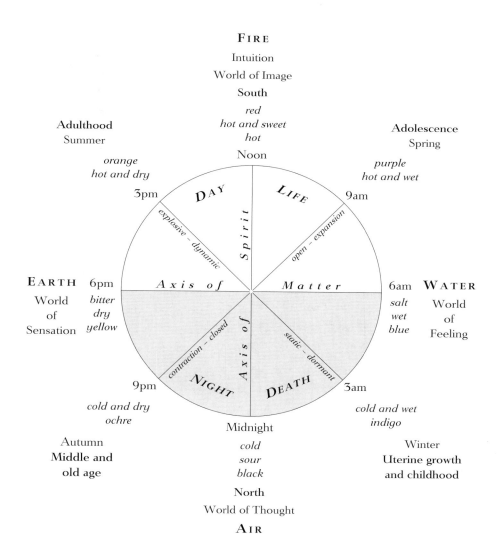

Fig. 9.2 a Mappa Mundi (after Misha Norland)[3] – the basic structure

THE HEAT PROCESS
Rejoicing and laughter.
Joy. Motivation.
Sublime trust. Love.

Brain.
Heart and arterial circulation.
Nervous system. Eyes and vision.
Sex and libido.

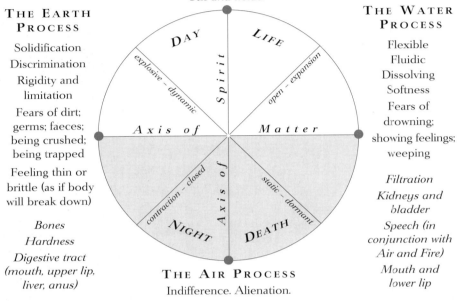

THE EARTH
PROCESS

Solidification
Discrimination
Rigidity and
limitation
Fears of dirt;
germs; faeces;
being crushed;
being trapped
Feeling thin or
brittle (as if body
will break down)

Bones
Hardness
Digestive tract
(mouth, upper lip,
liver, anus)

THE WATER
PROCESS

Flexible
Fluidic
Dissolving
Softness
Fears of
drowning;
showing feelings;
weeping

Filtration
Kidneys and
bladder
Speech (in
conjunction with
Air and Fire)
Mouth and
lower lip

THE AIR PROCESS
Indifference. Alienation.
Suicidal despair.
Fears of suffocation; falling; night; darkness;
death; damnation; evil; the devil; ghosts.
< Full moon
"The Dark Night of the Soul"

Oxidation and acidity. Lungs. Ears.
Sound. Cold reason and logic. Communication.

Fig. 9.2 b Mappa Mundi (after Misha Norland)[3] – the element correspondences

CHOLERIC
Dynamic and Forceful Characters

Irritable. Decisive. Explosive rages.
Formal. Intolerant of contradiction.
Aggressive. Accumulative.
Courageous. >Activity.

Yellow gall. Ducts in liver.
Bilirubin in blood. Stomach.
Inflammatory processes.

Hot dry earth –
lava, kiln, furnace,
oven.

SANGUINE
Sociable and Open Characters

Chatty. Bouncy. Childlike. Innocent.
Optimistic. Fear of loneliness.
Jealousy. >Discharges. >Company.

Blood and heart and arteries.
Skeletal muscles. Spleen. Dilation.
Congestion. Haemorrhage.

Hot and wet –
tropical rain forest,
steam, geysers.

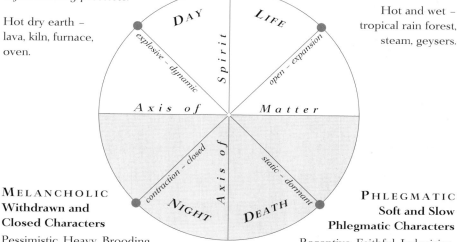

MELANCHOLIC
Withdrawn and
Closed Characters

Pessimistic. Heavy. Brooding.
Repressed. Restrained.
Feels ugly and worthless. Fear of loss.
Shuns company. Philosophical.
Introspective. Detached. Wise.
> Solitude.

Black Bile. Liver. Colon. Constipation.
Marasmus. Atrophy.

Cold dry earth – moon, steppes of
Central Asia.

PHLEGMATIC
Soft and Slow
Phlegmatic Characters

Receptive. Faithful. Indecisive.
Fear of domination; being engulfed.
Craving security and order.
Fears of loss of identity; loss of shape;
loss of structure. > Rest.

Lymphatic System. Synovial membranes.
Capsules. Cartilage. Conjunctivae.
Tears. Dropsy. Waterlogging.
Rheumatism. Phlegm.

Cold water – oceanic depths, mist, ice.

Fig. 9.2 c Mappa Mundi (after Misha Norland)[3] – the temperament correspondences

Remedies

Bryonia

We know that Bryonia is dry, irritable and doesn't want to move. The dryness relates it to the earth phase of the cycle (Bryonia has great thirst). This is confirmed by the fact that Bryonia is concerned with material safety and security – talks of business; fear of poverty; desires to go home. Dryness and inflammation (Bryonia is homœopathic to inflammation of any organ if the characteristic symptoms are present) point to the hot dry upper left quadrant. Bryonia has a 3pm aggravation (upper left quadrant). It also has a 3am aggravation, which is the place of stasis (lower right quadrant, polar opposite of upper left). Bryonia wants to be busy and industrious – upper left quadrant, choleric – and in their illness has to keep still, corresponding to the lower right quadrant.

Bryonia is very well known for its 9pm aggravation – the cold dry lower left quadrant. What can we make of this? This is the quadrant of the closed, withdrawn melancholic. Bryonia is "taciturn." "Wants to be alone; aversion to company as it causes one to talk and that means motion." There is "despair of being cured, and fear of death." "Very morose, ill-humoured."[4]

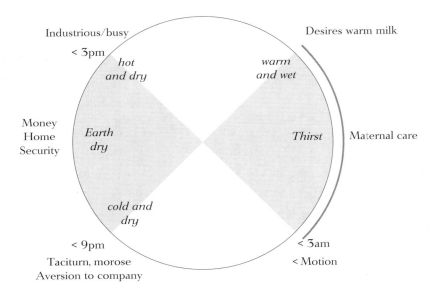

Fig. 9.3 Bryonia alba

< worse for   < better for

Bryonia has many symptoms concerned with the giving and receiving of milk – desire or aversion for milk, problems with lactation, mastitis. There is even "desire for warm milk".[5] This is surely an expression of the infant's longing for maternal warmth and security. Warm milk – warm and wet – would correspond to the upper right quadrant, the place of infancy and childhood, still within the sphere of maternal protection. "During delirium the patient expresses a continual 'desire to go home'; he imagines he is not at home and longs to be taken there in order to be properly taken care of." [6] This is the polar opposite of the cold, dry lower left quadrant that corresponds with 9pm.

Thus the themes of earth, mother and security are seen to be important in the remedy. The sense of insecurity makes Bryonia concerned with money and business. Always active and busy until, in their illness, they can't move. The inability to move faces them with their sense of lack of security and maternal warmth. If these feelings can be consciously faced, healing can come about. If not, the body carries the problem in the form of a Bryonia physical pathology.

Bryonia has a relationship to Natrum muriaticum, also known for dryness and mother issues.

Natrum muriaticum

Natrum muriaticum is associated with fluids and tears. It has a desire for or aversion to salt. All this places it in the water phase of the circle opposite Bryonia.

They are hopeful romantics who long for a deep relationship. Thus they are also susceptible to grief and disappointment from loss of the loved one. They can become melancholic (lower left quadrant), dry (cannot cry, cannot pass urine in presence of others, dry mucous membranes) and bitter (the taste associated with the dry earth phase). Hopeful yearning for romantic attachment is easily disappointed and they become emotionally walled off, melancholic, harbouring bitter resentments. Often the relationship with their mother was disappointing. They wanted her affection but may have perceived her as cold or distant (cold and dry, lower left quadrant).

The remedy is well known for its 10am aggravation (almost opposite the 9pm of Bryonia). This confirms it to be on the axis between upper right and lower left quadrant. This is also the axis of open and closed. They opened to love and were hurt. He or she becomes closed and withdrawn. They feel worse from sympathy because this activates old hurts (these are like the salt crystals that are no longer in solution!). They feel things will never be right (rubric: grief for the future – also melancholic), although they secretly yearn for love, falling in love with unobtainable people (such as a married man or woman). In this way they can return, in their imagination, to the hopeful springtime of new romance.

Symbolically we might think of the remedy as being like the salt crystal, which, as it were, wants to become an individual crystal while at the same time wishing to dissolve back into the ocean from which it came. As a dynamic symbol, this corresponds to the emergence of the emotional/feeling self that we discussed in chapters three and four. In this stage of development the self must break the symbiotic union with the mother so that it can continue to grow and individuate.

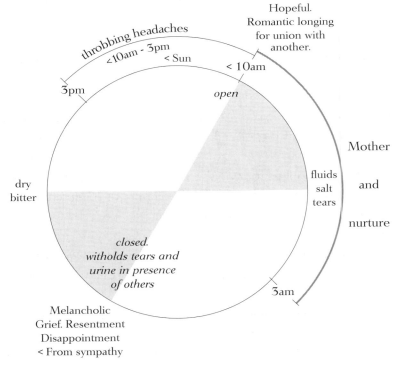

Fig. 9.4 Natrum muriaticum

The individual who needs Natrum muriaticum is especially sensitive to this conflict (between symbiotic union and individuality). Thus they seek affection (rubric: affectionate) and reject it at the same time (rubric: consolation aggravates). It is as though they are torn between the need for intimate union (oceanic) and the need to be a separate individual (the salt crystal).[7]

Someone who has a problem rooted in this developmental stage will have a problem with the making and breaking of the relationship with the mother, and thus with the making and breaking of all subsequent intimate relationships.

What can be made of the well-known aggravation from the sun found in this remedy? There are throbbing, pounding headaches, worse from the sun and worse between 10am and 3pm. Symbolically speaking the sun calls you into activity and engagement with life. It calls you to individuation and self-consciousness. To go forward in life the Natrum muriaticum individual must let go of the past and stop dwelling on old grievances. They must learn to be an individual, but not walled off from the flow of life and relationship.

Belladonna and Calcarea carbonica
The figures overleaf illustrate the inner dynamics of Belladonna and Calcarea carbonica.

In Belladonna there is a particular emphasis on fire. There is "heat, redness, throbbing and burning."[8] There is "violence of attack, and suddenness of onset". Even to extremes – "furious; rages, bites, strikes". There are "visions of fire" and there is "fury and heat of the body". The remedy is focused in the hot and dry quadrant (upper left – opposite Calcarea carbonica). "Burning heat, bright redness and dryness are very marked."[9] There is a marked 3pm aggravation. In opposition to this (opposite quadrant) there is an "abhorrence of liquids."[10]

There is also much that belongs to the night realm (lower quadrant of the circle). Here, as we shall see, it coincides with Calcarea. At the nadir of the circle, 12 midnight, we encounter a cold dark airless realm, opposite the heat and light found at the zenith of the circle. Belladonna "imagines he sees ghosts, hideous faces, and various insects; black animals, dogs, wolves, etc.". The patient (or prover) "imagines himself dreaming when awake", and "sees faces on closing the eyes" or has "horrible visions in the dark."[11] The psyche is

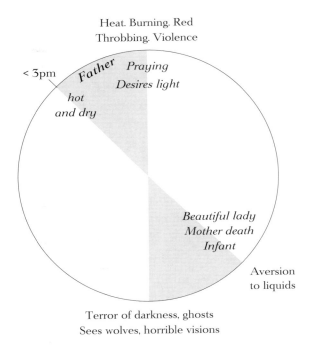

Heat. Burning. Red
Throbbing. Violence

< 3pm

Father *Praying*

Desires light

hot
and dry

Beautiful lady
Mother death
Infant

Aversion
to liquids

Terror of darkness, ghosts
Sees wolves, horrible visions

Fig. 9.5 Belladonna

invaded by unconscious terrors and images of the night. Thus there is also
desire for light and praying (zenith of the circle).

In this remedy we find terror, rage and the need to flee. Primal feelings
break free from conscious controls. Thus it is a remedy of infancy, feverish
delirium and drug or alcohol induced states – all conditions in which conscious controls are reduced.

Belladonna is particularly known as an infants remedy. Sankaran writes,
"The main feeling of a Belladonna person is of a sudden threat from outside from
which he has to escape in order to survive." [12] In terms of developmental stages
this feeling would be most typical in infancy. It is in the earliest stages of life
that threat to existence (or the feeling of threat to existence) can be most acute.

With this in mind the various names of the plant are revealing. In psychology much has been made of the infant's experience of the good mother
and the bad mother. From a psychological point of view the infant perceives
himself to be surrounded by archetypal forces (in the form of the parents), at

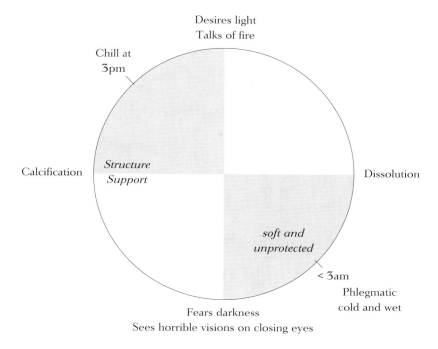

Fig. 9.6 Calcarea carbonica

once loving and terrible. For the infant the presence of the mother summons the presence of the "archetypal" mother – the one who, in the primitive imagination of the infant, is the great source of nourishment and love, and, in her anger or indifference, also the possible source of abandonment, destruction and death. She is the "beautiful lady" (bella donna) who can also be the terrible "mother death" (Nah-Skado – the goddess from whose name the word "nightshade" may be derived).[13] With this talk of the mother, what of the father? The young child needs the presence and guidance of male energy (fire, father, drive, structure, upper half of the circle) to help him or her to separate from the hold of the mother. The male influence in the life of the child can of course also be experienced as positive or detrimental.

Calcarea carbonica belongs to the phlegmatic quadrant (lower right – cold and wet). The patient is "fat, fair, flabby and perspiring and cold, damp and sour". We read, "children who grow fat, are large bellied, with large head, pale skin, chalky look, the so called leucophlegmatic temperament". There is "perspiration, especially about the head, feet and hands." There is "tardy teething and late walking". Muscles are easily strained. Calcarea individuals are said to be "slow conscientious workers who steadily plod along." [14] Thus, "it is very useful in complaints from prolonged worry, from prolonged application to business, from excitement." [15] The patient feels vulnerable, without protection and support (the oyster shell). The patient feels that they could break down under stress.

There is lack of a shell to protect from the world. They need to be at home (repertory: home, desires to go). They feel vulnerable and are badly affected by the thought of cruelty or harm to others. They can also feel observed and criticised.

It is as though there is also lack of mental structure to protect from the images and darkness of the unconscious. There is anxiety at twilight, aggravation from darkness, and so on. Like Belladonna, the patient "sees visions on closing the eyes." The child sees and fears monsters and horrible things. "Children with night terrors, waking at 3am." [16] This 3am aggravation (lower right quadrant) is opposite the 3pm of Belladonna. Given all this, it isn't surprising that "fear of madness" is a marked symptom of Calcarea carbonica.

The homœopathic masters of the past recognised Belladonna as the acute of Calcarea carbonica. Calcarea stands for passive withdrawal and need for protection. Belladonna stands for active "fight or flight" in the face of sudden threat.

In conclusion

You could take almost any remedy and put the main symptoms on the circle. This will usually give insight into the unified pattern that underlies the symptom picture of the remedy. You can also of course use the map as an aid to understanding the pattern behind the diverse symptoms present in a patient.

In the symbolism of the Mappa Mundi, each person has tendencies to certain weaknesses and disorders. These are defined by temperament and constitution. A person tends towards the phlegmatic, choleric, sanguine or melancholic. They are constituted in certain proportions of fire, air, water and earth. They will lean towards the disorders associated with these elements and temperaments.

The map also helps one to understand polarity and compensation. If there is over emphasis in one direction, the self-righting function of the vital force attempts to rectify the balance by accentuating the opposite polarity. If there is too much dryness for example, the denied water element will appear somewhere else, perhaps in the form of watery discharges. The overly responsible Aurum patient, who could plunge down into the depths of suicidal despair, also suffers from "vertigo in high places." In Aurum there is a conflict between height of achievement and duty, and depth of despair.

You have, we might say, a place on the circle that is at once your wound and your opportunity. It's the place where your rhythm and adaptability tend to get stuck with the subsequent fall into polarity and conflict. In sickness one is pulled apart by opposites. One is in a state of conflict. In healing it is necessary to find a new centre of gravity that transcends and includes the conflicting tendencies within oneself.[17]

The ancient Chinese philosophers suggested that the work of man is to adapt his activity to the seasonal flow of time. In this way the twin principles of consciousness and nature are brought together to the benefit of both nature and consciousness. Lets finish this chapter with advice from the I Ching on harmonising these two primary spheres of human makeup. The Richard Wilhelm translation of the I Ching puts it beautifully in hexagram 11, *peace*.

Heaven and earth are in contact and combine their influences, producing a time of universal flowering and prosperity. This stream of energy must be regulated by the ruler of men *[i.e. your own inner understanding and authority]*. It is done by a process of division. Thus men divide the uniform flow of time into the seasons, according to the succession of natural phenomena, and mark off infinite space by points of the compass. In this way nature in its overwhelming profusion of phenomena is bounded and controlled. On the other hand, nature must be furthered in her productiveness. This is done by adjusting the products to the right time and the right place, which increases the natural yield. This controlling and furthering activity of man in his relation to nature is the work on nature that rewards him.[18]

In other words our task is to bring our consciousness into harmonious relationship with all that is natural and good both in and around us.

Chapter 10:
Similarity

In this chapter I want to look at the significance and use of the principle of similarity. Homœopaths have long held that this principle deserves to be considered as a law of nature. It should, they say, be thought of as a natural law alongside others, like gravity or magnetism for example. At any rate the experience of homœopaths over the last two hundred years testifies to the fact that similarity is a fundamental principle of healing.

In this chapter I'll suggest that similarity is, first and foremost, a general principle of consciousness concerned with recognition and memory. It is in fact on this basis that it is also a law of healing. Healing is, in a certain sense, a re-cognition or a re-membering. What it is exactly that has to be re-membered we'll come to shortly.

First a little about similarity as a scientific principle. The science of similarity is the science of resonance. All non-physical forces, like sound or electricity, have waves that oscillate at certain frequencies. Frequencies in one field of activity can produce effects in another field of activity. According to scientific theory when any system capable of oscillating, a tuning fork for example, is excited by another oscillating system (like another vibrating tuning fork), waves are excited in the original system. In other words at the vibrational level things that are similar resonate together, like two similarly tuned strings.[1]

Let's now consider the idea of similarity a little further. First the meaning of the word "similar". It refers to things that resemble each other in appearance, form, qualities, characteristics, and so on. We use similarity to recognise things in relation to one another.

For example if you look at a drawing of someone you know, even a simple line drawing like a cartoon, you immediately know who the drawing represents. Even a few lines on a piece of paper can be enough to evoke recognition of that person. This occurs through the principle of similarity. The line drawing is not an identical representation of the face, but it has to be similar enough, particularly in bringing out the characteristic features (like a cartoon), to bring about recognition.

Memory itself also uses the principle of similarity of one whole to another. When you see or experience something, similar experiences are brought forward from your memory. The drawing evokes, through similarity, the memory of the person represented. In the study of memory this is called pattern recognition. Pattern recognition occurs when a match is made between incoming sensory information and a pattern of data in the long-term memory system.[2]

Before going on let's look at some examples of similarity as a general principle of life and consciousness. In doing this I'll be taking a lead from Hahnemann who, in his *Organon of the Medical Art,* sites a number of instances of cure through the natural occurrence of the law of similarity.[3] I hope these examples will help us to understand similarity as a law of consciousness concerned with memory and recognition. Then we'll look at how homœopathy makes therapeutic use of this law.

Similarity in life

In Chapter one I mentioned morphic fields. The morphic field of an organism structures its form and programs its functions. Rupert Sheldrake suggests that the morphic field of an organism relates to the physical aspect of the organism through morphic resonance. He suggests that the "recognition" between organism and morphogenetic field takes place through similar rhythmic activity in both vibrational field and physical organism. Through similarity the organism is able to respond to the information coded in the frequencies of its morphic field.[4]

In a similar vein Jung describes what happens when typical life situations – love, achievement, conflict, and so on – are encountered. When such an encounter occurs a similar archetypal imprint is awakened. A deeply rooted pattern of behaviour is activated. Thus, in love, courtship behaviour is awoken. This behaviour comes from a universal pattern that has been replayed and reinforced countless times in the history of the species. This activation of the archetype happens because of the similarity of the particular life situation to the related collective memory and experience of humanity.[5] This archetypal response is both psychological and biological.

Here's a fascinating story illustrating another aspect of similarity. It's reported by Joseph Campbell from an account given by the famous explorer Leo Frobenius.[6] The explorer was in Africa and asked a group of natives who accompanied his party to find and kill an antelope for the kitchen. They told him preparations were needed and they would not be able to hunt until the following day. He was intrigued to know what preparations these might be. He was amazed to discover that they consisted of the tribesmen drawing an antelope in the sand in a spot at which they had gathered before sunrise. At the moment of sunrise, to the accompaniment of ritual incantations, the image was ceremoniously shot through the neck, whereupon the men ran off into the forest. Later that day the men returned to the camp kitchen with an antelope – shot through the neck.

The whole and the part

In these examples we can see that it is necessary for the part to be in harmony with a higher order, a more embracing whole. The functioning of the individual butterfly has to be attuned to the collective morphic field of butterflies on which its form and function is dependent.

In human life our individual actions take their cue from larger collective patterns or archetypes. Individual feelings and reactions occur within the context of deeper, older and more powerful collective patterns. When we love we enact the drama of all lovers, of love itself. Problems arise when archetypal responses are active without our awareness. It is only when we remain mindful that we can be aware of the activity of these powers within us. This mindfulness – this remembering – makes it possible for unconscious, and thus often negative and destructive, patterns of feeling and behaviour to become more conscious. When this happens it is less likely that energy will flow into negative or destructive habits. This means that energy becomes less bound, freer. In other words we become less confined by habitual responses and more able to be creatively in the present.

The antelope hunters had to attune themselves to the "great spirit" of the antelope. By their "similarity ritual" they attuned themselves to the collective spirit of antelope (today we would say morphic field). Through the spiritual intent of their ritual the gift of the antelope was asked for.[7]

Holons

We understood in Chapter 1 that holons have some fundamental, and universally present, characteristics. Among the most important of these is that all holons are part/wholes. They are wholes made of parts, and are also part of larger wholes (atoms, molecules, cells, organs, creatures, planet, solar system, and so on). For a holon such as the human to be healthy, its parts need to function in harmonious integration. It also needs to be a harmonious part of a greater whole. So the human being needs to be in a state of internal integration, as well as being connected to (integrated into) a greater whole (family, culture, the life of the Earth, the life of spirit, and so on).

Human beings need to feel themselves as part of something greater that embodies a vision of the meaning, purpose and possibilities of life. Such a vision has always been embodied in the many and varied religious approaches to life, which formed the heart of all cultures in the past. Without this connection to community, and beyond community, to an all-embracing holy vision of life and the human being's role in it, life becomes a desert and the soul shrivels and dies.

Disease, forgetting and remembering

Let's return to the question of disease and remembering. What, in disease, is it that has been forgotten, and what has to be remembered in order to restore health?

We have seen how the emergence of human self-consciousness, while an absolutely necessary development, also ruptures the primal wholeness of being. This is true both in the development of the infant from birth, and, on the larger historical canvas, the development of the particularly self-conscious thinking human being out of the matrix of human prehistory. Thus it is necessary to continually remind ourselves of whom we truly are – that is, whole and complete parts of a larger whole (culture, earth, spirit, etc.). It is the strangest of paradoxes that in becoming conscious human beings forget their true nature and true belonging. And yet it is only through becoming conscious that we can truly know who we are and the great mystery of which we are a part.

This reminding activity was given the greatest importance in cultures of the past. In the distant past, those individuals charged with a special responsibility for human society and culture instituted a cycle of rituals which were intended to repair the damage to the fabric of cosmos, earth and human nature caused by the emerging presence of human consciousness. The purpose of these rituals, seasonally enacted, was to reveal to the participants, as though in a mirror (in other words, through similarity), the true nature of the human condition. These rituals reminded the participants of the nature of their loss and suffering, their loss of wholeness, and helped to bring about a remembering of their true and always present nature. It was a profound and timely reminder of the oneness of all life and of the one spirit behind all manifestation.[8]

Symptoms

But what of the individual's loss of wholeness and need for re-integration? How does homœopathy address this? In disease, sensations and dysfunctions that most especially draw our attention by virtue of their uncomfortable presence are the symptoms that constitute the homœopathic totality. They represent the parts that are out of harmony with the whole. They are thus also the parts that cry out for integration. These parts of ourselves may appear as images, as troublesome feelings, or unpleasant sensations (as well as dysfunctions of one sort or another). They are the messengers of dismembered wholeness.

When a similar remedy is presented to the disturbed wholeness of the patient – manifest in the totality of characteristic symptoms – it quiets those parts of wholeness (the symptoms) that have fallen out of harmony and thus, like ignored children, cry out to be heard. Surely it quiets them because they are now, as it were, heard and recognised? The remedy heals through the power of recognition and acceptance. The remedy shows the psyche how things are (similarity) rather than attempting to drive the suffering parts away (contra).

Of course the healing capacity of the similar remedy can only come into play on the basis of the capacity of the homœopath to recognise and accept what is suffering and unintegrated within the patient. Without the recognition by the homœopath of what cries out to be heard in the patient, the similimum cannot be given. Furthermore the homœopath can only recognise the nature of this suffering when the patient can freely speak of it. Thus the remedy is the child of the exchange between patient and homœopath. Sometimes this exchange will be graced by understanding and insight and sometimes not. A deep-acting similimum is only ever given when understanding has clicked and when all the elements of the case are seen to fall into a consistent pattern.

In healing, what was troublesome finds its place again. Where the part had ruled our consciousness – with good reason, because it had become an excluded part – there is now a kind of emptiness in which new possibilities can bud and flower. Where the part had cried out for attention there is now a "nothing in particular" which we might call "no-thing-ness." What one does with this nothingness after the gift of homœopathy has brought the parts back into harmony is of course an open question. We are free to enjoy this freedom. We are free to be in a state of joy rather than ruled by the polarities of pleasure and pain. It all depends on whether we are ready for the emptiness of freedom and the freedom of emptiness.

Similarity and Susceptibility

The notion of similarity leads us to a closely related idea, that of susceptibility. To be susceptible to something means to be easily influenced by it. The word comes from the Latin meaning "to undertake." This suggests that being susceptible to an influence means you take it on, you bear it, you suffer it. A person can be susceptible to ideas, people, diseases, and so on. If a person is, for example, susceptible to tuberculosis they undertake the condition of tuberculosis.

It is susceptibility that decides if I succumb to this or that virus or bacteria. It decides which weather conditions, foods, people and events that I am particularly influenced by.

Hahnemann suggests that susceptibility arises from a "mistunement" of the vital force whereby a particular influence can become a "morbific influence". Any influence, whether physical or psychic can, according to him, become a "disease potence" if susceptibility is present.[9] A potence is a dynamic field of influence that may or may not take a physical form. So a potence could be a bacteria, a thought, a feeling, a climatic condition, a food, even a time of day. A potence could be inside me or outside me. It could be another person or a piece of music. It could be a thought, feeling or image that I carry within myself.

When a person is especially attuned to such a dynamic field they become particularly sensitive to its influence. If I am attuned to the flu virus, or to hot weather, or to darkness, these things can become "morbific" influences rather than ordinary events. They become disease potences. In other words I get flu, or tend to become overheated, or am fearful in the dark. A disease potence is a morphic field to which a person is particularly attuned and thus is especially sensitive to. This sensitivity makes the person vulnerable to its influence. They easily let it in. They easily undertake it.

Let's look at this in a slightly different way. Clearly sensitivity is not in itself a bad thing. In fact it is the spice of life. We are moved in a creative way by music, art, landscape, the presence of another person. However, certain things, situations or conditions will touch us in such a way that the sensitivity becomes, as it were, a painful sensitivity. The influence becomes a "disease potence." This happens when something vulnerable and protected is being touched. Sometimes this is fine, as when we cry at a moving scene in a film.

So what is happening when a sensitivity of some kind becomes problematic? What happens when a sensitivity – to food, people, events, weather, a time of day – frequently produces a problem in physical or psychological health? What might lie behind such a sensitivity?

An environmental condition to which I have a special morbid sensitivity – flu, heat, darkness, a certain kind of person, a certain landscape – highlights what is unacknowledged and unintegrated in myself. What do I mean by this? Someone is sensitive to a particular influence because it touches some aspect of them that is particularly reactive. So why are they reactive in this way? They are reactive to this influence because it corresponds to something unmet and unintegrated within them. They are sensitive and unguarded against the out-side influence because it is *similar* to a place of difficulty within them. This place of difficulty is a place of poor adaptation. It is a place where life is stuck. (We have seen that all "intake" – solids, liquids, gases, sensory experience, emotional experience – has to be assimilated and integrated. If food is not assimilated the rhythm of digestion can be disturbed. If experiences are not integrated the rhythm of the soul is blocked or upset.)

Susceptibility is present when the outer situation reminds the psyche of what is incomplete or undigested within. When the organism is faced with assimilating something (experiencing something, taking something in) that is similar to something that is, so to speak, already in the system but unintegrated or "undigested", then there is a reaction. This sensitivity, because it is uncon-scious and unrecognised, may well take the form of a physical sensitivity.

Let's take an example. A person feels worse at twilight (a feeling of unease provoked by a sensory experience of fading light associated with the decline of the day). The external condition of twilight aggravates something "twilight like" in the person. At twilight one stands, as it were, on the edge of your own inner darkness. For some this is a pleasant experience, a time of relaxation and peace. For others – those who need remedies such as Phos-phorus or Calcarea carbonica – the onset of darkness awakens the terror and uncertainty of an inner darkness. There is a resonance – a similarity – between the outer condition and an area of unconscious difficulty within the patient. (Resonance can occur between any physical or non-physical pres-ence, because everything, physical and non-physical, has a field – thus the sensory condition of low light can resonate with, and thus awaken, a psycho-logical feeling of fear or abandonment.) The condition of low light awakens early (infant, child) experiences of darkness, aloneness and abandonment that have not been integrated. These experiences remain unconscious, repressed and unassimilated. They remain as sticking points in the flow of life.

Inner and outer

The notion of susceptibility raises a further important point. When I fall prey to flu, I don't talk about "my" flu virus, I say "the" flu virus. I recognise that the flu virus is out there in the environment, and that through my susceptibility it has been able to gain an entrance. However, when we talk of fear or anger we adopt a rather different stance. We say my fear or my anger, as though the fear or anger was ours. We could however think about this in a different way. If I am susceptible to anger, it means that I undertake anger. This suggests that anger, like the flu virus, is an objective entity to which I become susceptible. Looked at like this, anger is no longer "my anger" but an objective power in the world to which I have become susceptible. Like the flu virus, it now lives in me. I then wrestle with it as something within me that must be got rid of. It is freeing to realise that it is not my anger, but anger itself. My responsibility does not concern anger itself, but my susceptibility to anger. Change that and anger can no longer take root. On a larger scale the less that anger itself can take root in the soil of individual souls, the less that the world power of anger itself can thrive and grow strong.[10]

Susceptibility and Consciousness

The nineteenth century American homœopath, J. T. Kent, used the rather curious term "susceptibility is satisfied."[11] He suggests that susceptibility must be satisfied if cure is to take place. What can we make of this strange statement in the light of what has already been said? The words suggest that susceptibility represents a need within us that wants to be met, needs to be satisfied. But a need for what?

Susceptibility exists where there is heightened sensitivity, heightened reactivity. We can also say that susceptibility exists where there is a need for healing. The need for healing exists where there is a need for change and greater awareness. This is a need for more inclusiveness and wholeness. There is a need to resolve and integrate an area of unconscious resistance and difficulty. Thus areas of vulnerability and sensitivity – sensitive and vulnerable because repressed or ignored – will be called forth, *through similarity*, by the conditions, events and people that are encountered in life.

In being called forth, these sensitivities offer a doorway into a more complete and integrated wholeness. It is the dynamic interaction between world (cause) and self (susceptibility) that points to the road of healing and wholeness.

Through susceptibility we respond to situations from a place of damaged sensitivity. But hidden in this response is a desire to be well and whole.

For this wellness to come about we need to refrain from trying to fix the apparent cause of suffering. Instead we need to look to the source of our susceptibility. In other words we need to be shown the nature of the wound, the nature of the problem within our own selves. This "showing", this recognition clears the "stuckness" of the vital force, and allows what was unintegrated to be re-integrated into the harmony of the whole. This is done through the mirror of similarity. When this happens the susceptibility, and the hidden desire for change and healing that is concealed within the susceptibility, is satisfied. The need for wholeness and healing, which secretly operates within our susceptibilities, is satisfied. In homœopathic treatment this happens when the remedy, in its potentised form, is similar to the unconscious dynamics of conflict which give rise to the form of the disease.

Chapter 11:
Provings

One of Hahnemann's gifts to medicine was the development of a method for establishing which remedial agents were similar to which disease symptoms. The methodology is well documented by Hahnemann himself, and more recently by such teachers as Jeremy Sherr.[1] Let's just remind ourselves. The method involves the testing of potentised substances on healthy human individuals. To this pure empirical data is added known toxicological data as well as clinical data from cured symptoms in practise.

Hahnemann didn't invent the idea of treatment by similars. However his new methodology was a significant step forward in the history of treatment by similars. Before this, physicians had relied on other less satisfactory methods to establish the link of similarity between medicine and patient. Physicians were guided by the doctrine of signatures. This teaching simply says that the essence or spirit of a plant can be seen in its form, colour, mode of growth, and so on. The great physician philosopher Paracelsus writes:

"There is nothing that Nature has not signed in such a way that man may discover its essence ... As you can see, each herb is given the form that befits its nature; similarly man is endowed with a form corresponding to his inner nature. And just as the form shows what a given herb is, so the human sign indicates what a given man is ... Since nothing is so secret or hidden that it cannot be revealed, everything depends on the discovery of those things which manifest the hidden ... For the sculptor of Nature is so artful that he does not fashion the soul to fit the form, but the form to fit the soul."[2]

So the essence of something is revealed in its form. According to the doctrine of signatures if something of the form of a plant, for example, is suggestive of or similar to a human function or pathology, then there is an inner connection between the two. Thus, for example, the yellow-flowered greater celandine was held to be useful in the treatment of jaundice – a fact that has been born out by homœopathic observation.

People in the past may, through natural intuition and the accumulated knowledge of natural healers, have been able to sense the connections between nature and human beings in a manner that to us moderns is a closed book. Take Pulsatilla as an example. One of its common names is "shame faced maiden." [3] From homœopathic clinical experience we know that the person who needs the remedy is timid, changeable, and can be shy of the opposite sex. They can even develop fixed ideas about religion and sex; they can become prone to religious dos and don'ts and believe that sex is sinful. "Shame faced maiden" seems strangely appropriate, but how was it so named before homœopathic provings revealed these characteristics of the remedy?

Rudolph Steiner, working from indications given by Goethe, suggested a similar approach, attempting to see a correspondence between the inner formative forces of a mineral or plant and the physical, psychological and spiritual functions of the human being in health and disease. [4] In this way it might be discovered which plant or mineral corresponds with which disease process, thus revealing its possible therapeutic value.

The weakness of this approach is that it is rather general and can lead to rather vague conclusions. Indeed Hahnemann is known to have dismissed the doctrine of signatures claiming that it gave rise to all kinds of unfounded and unscientific speculations. [5] I'm going to suggest a kinder point of view, which is this. Hahnemann took the essential idea of the doctrine of signatures – that is, the attempt to understand the similarity between the remedial agent and the disease condition to be treated – and combined it with the rigorousness of the newly discovered empirical science of his day to produce an empirical method which honoured both old and new approaches. Thus through provings we discover, through a scientific method, the mark or signature of the remedial substance in its relation to human constitution. Paracelsus had already pointed the way; "everything depends on the discovery of those things which manifest the hidden." It was another three centuries before Hahnemann would come up with a scientific solution to the dilemma posed by his great predecessor.

As a matter of fact homœopaths often compliment their understanding of the provings with data drawn from the signature of the substance as it is traditionally or symbolically understood. Thus when we recall the association of Sulphur, not only with volcanoes but – symbolically – with fire and brimstone, hell and damnation, we are not surprised to find along with the sensations of heat and burning, all kinds of thoughts and feelings associated with a "fall from grace" – the belief that he was disgraced (repertory: delusion, she is disgraced), fear of poverty and even a fear of heights (symbolic of the fear of an inner fall). The prover of Lac canninum, dog bitch's milk, feels dirty and inferior, revealing exactly how our inner "bitch" nature feels when we mistreat and ignore it, or when we are maltreated by others. The person who needs Argentum metallicum (silver) is concerned with image and performance. They attempt to reflect the expected image back to the world. The signature of silver lies in its use in mirrors and light sensitive photographic paper, as well as its traditional association with the moon (which reflects solar light).

A word of warning here. If we try and anticipate the results of a proving through an interpretation of the already known data (scientific, traditional or symbolic data related to a mineral, plant or animal), we will easily come unstuck. The first task of a proving is to establish the pure and uninterpreted data. Only when this has been established and been put to the test in clinical practise can we allow ourselves to see whether this data seems to confirm the ideas and physical properties that are already associated with the substance. It is well here to recall Hahnemann's injunctions about unnecessary speculation.[6]

The proving experience

A proving should give subjective and objective data (the inside and outside of the human holon). Thus a well-documented proving consists of a montage of thoughts, feelings, images and physical sensations experienced by the prover, along with observable changes in behaviour and bodily function.

Potency

If the inner nature of a substance is to be understood, it must be proved in potency. Crude substance produces crude effects (poisonings). Potentisation releases the formative, the "idea" within substance. Thus a proving with a potentised substance awakens the formative within the prover. It is the psyche that responds to the potency, just as the body responds to substance.

Furthermore, according to Hahnemann, the essence of disease is "spirit like", invisible, psychic. It thus needs to be met by something vital, dynamic and "spirit like". Put another way, what is psychological in origin (disease) needs to be met by the psychic dimension of a remedial substance. This psychic dimension is set free through potentisation. It is this that acts therapeutically, and this that needs to be experienced by a prover. The homœopathic prover becomes attuned to the "spirit" of the substance. This is rather like a radio being tuned to a particular broadcast frequency. The prover is in a sense taken over by the frequency of the substance, thus giving a human expression to the characteristics and properties of the potence in question.

The potentised proving substance can be thought of as the memory or imprint of a power (plant, animal etc.) of nature. It is not that power itself, but a bridge to that power. Just as a photograph can evoke the presence of a real person, and a recording can evoke the presence of musicians, so the potentised remedy can evoke the presence of a power of nature (the spirit of plant, animal or mineral).

The imprint or memory that is the potence evokes something similar from that world of archetypal energies which lies at the root of the prover's constitution, the world of "nature" within the prover. This experience may be pleasant or unpleasant. Let's look at this a little more closely.

Primary and secondary action

We have already looked at polarity in disease. Hahnemann maintained that polarities could also be observed in provings. He established that provings consist of a primary action and a secondary action. The first is the action of the potence on the vital force of the prover, and the second is the reaction of the vital force.[7] If, for example, a potence produces a primary action of sleepiness, then the secondary action will be wakefulness. In practise things aren't as cut and dry as this. Action and reaction follow one another in cyclic

186

fashion. Conditions within the prover will predispose the prover to one polarity or other of the proving effect. Thus one prover may experience joy, and another sorrow. Yet another will experience joy followed by sorrow, and so on.[8]

All kinds of images, thoughts, feelings and sensations could appear in the first stages of the proving. However it is not unusual for some kind of "high" to be the first sign that an alteration in the awareness and the vital force of the prover is occurring. The prover may laugh, feel good, have significant insights or other forms of "peak experience."[9] This is the primary action. It is as though the potency, in that it has been released from matter, represents a kind of freedom from gravity and matter and thus awakens in the prover a similar sense of spiritual release.

Sooner or later, whatever the initial experiences may be, secondary symptoms appear. These are the reaction of mind and body attempting to come to terms with the "alien" presence of remedy field. The vital force reacts to the field of the substance. This is something like having to assimilate and adapt to an unforeseen experience. It is as though a "spirit" in the form of an idea or image had taken hold of one's being. The psyche must accommodate its presence.

Integration

In the human individual the presence of the potence has to be integrated. Once it has entered it must in some way be processed. The experience to be assimilated is the same in different provers. However, the reactions of the provers vary, just as different people will have different reactions to a particular person although they will all recognise that it is the same person.

Hence, in provings, different constitutions will respond in different ways. There are a number of factors to be considered here. Is the prover easily overwhelmed or not, easily influenced or not? What about their sense of identity? Is that sound or fragile? Are they a strongly defended personality or not? Are they psychologically well integrated? There may be unrecognised or unhealed trauma. Physical health is another consideration. Vital organs may be healthy or weak. The body may already be struggling with toxicity. To what extent have chronic disorders taken hold? Inherited weaknesses may have compromised the ability to react and adapt.

If the prover is relatively free of baggage, is not carrying too much un-digested shadow material either personal or ancestral, and is relatively free of physical toxicity, then the potence will pass through the being of the prover without much upset. However if there is trauma or conflict related to early development or there are deep rooted ancestral patterns of disease in mind or body, or there is physical toxicity, then the channels of psychological and physical functioning will be constricted, blocked with debris or otherwise dys-functional. Then the proving may be long and arduous and the process of integration full of struggle.[10]

In provings, as in life, it is often the resistance to what are felt to be dif-ficult or painful experiences that cause more problems than the experiences themselves. In provings, as in life, all experiences need to be processed and integrated. If there is a capacity to open to the experiences, the painful as well as the pleasurable, then things will not be so bad. It's better to enter willingly into an inevitable experience, rather than be forced into it. It is better to surf the wave than try and swim against it. When resistance arises, for whatever reason, to the presence of the potence, there will be difficulty. In any event there is bound to be a measure of resistance because the prover inevitably encounters something new, and thus even in a healthy prover there will be the challenge of the unknown and the need to integrate the new and unex-pected.

Thus after the initial effects we are likely to see the downside of the proving kicking in. There could be any of the whole range of human fears and painful or difficult feelings, such as suspicion, anger, loneliness, despair. These may arise with accompanying thoughts, images and sensations. When the inner experiences induced by the proving cannot be integrated, the problem resonates in the body and we see the emergence of physical symptoms. Var-ious pains and alterations in body function will probably occur at some stage. The various changes experienced by the prover don't necessarily follow one another in orderly sequence. One prover will reflect one polarity of the potence, another prover the other polarity. One prover will experience more psychological changes, and another physical, and in others more of the whole picture will be seen.

Provings are analogous to disease

Hahnemann thought of provings as artificially induced disease processes.[11] In other words the process of a proving is analogous to the process of disease. Lets consider this further.

A proving is an encounter with a "power" of nature in the form of the potence. The presence of the potence arouses reaction as the self, in both its psychological and physical aspects, attempts to accommodate this presence. In life also there is a need to assimilate many and diverse influences (potences); those of micro-organisms, weather conditions, foods, feelings, thoughts, other people, culture, to name but a few. The activity of assimilation may be trouble free, or may be felt as disturbing. The process of assimilation of influences comes to us in the form of our reactions – thoughts, feelings, sensations, changes in function, and so on.

In life whatever enters the field of awareness or the physical body needs to be processed and integrated, whether we are willing or not. Sometimes we have the capacity to accept these influences and at other times not. An influence that is felt to be painful or unacceptable will naturally be resisted. Difficulty in acceptance and assimilation, whether of a psychological or physical influence, constitutes the presence of illness. If we eat something bad, for example, then there is indigestion until the body has assimilated or discharged the noxious substance. Likewise, grief may lie heavily until the experience is fully assimilated.

In a proving, primary symptoms are followed by secondary symptoms. These are the symptoms of an "artificial disease." Once the influence of the potence has been accepted, integrated and discharged, the artificial disease ends.

Acute and chronic

There is an important difference between the proving situation and general life situations. By and large, provings are self-limiting and life situations are chronic. Let's consider this important and fundamental difference.

A proving is a direct and rapid confrontation with a power. In this sense it is closer to an acute disease. In an acute illness the immune system is temporarily, and more or less rapidly, placed under great stress or threat. It may even be overwhelmed, with fatal consequences. The response, especially in children, is inflammation and fever.

Together with the immune response the psyche may also be threatened or overwhelmed. For example fever can be accompanied by delirium and unusual states of mind. In these states unconscious realms of the imagination become more visible. For example a child who needs Belladonna is beset by images of monsters.

It isn't only fevers that can produce this state of affairs. Febrile states have something in common with acute manias, poisoning by plant alkaloids or animal proteins, as well as drug or alcohol induced states. In all these conditions, as well as immune reaction, conscious controls are temporally overwhelmed. Powerful delusions and affects, usually kept in check by the conscious self, are able to surface.

In these situations the immune system together with normal conscious controls are stressed or overwhelmed. Thus along with immune response (inflammation, etc.) unbridled impulse and delusion are more able to surface. Balance is restored when the immune system and/or the conscious personality is able to re-establish the status quo.

A proving is another instance of more or less acute reaction. (Although of course some proving symptoms can be very long lasting; the proving can become a chronic disease). The sudden presence of the proving potence overwhelms the normal conscious controls in the manner described above. For example the proving of Aurum metallicum produces a desire for suicide. Although this is a key symptom of Aurum, there will be Aurum patients who are not suicidal. The patient who needs Aurum will have learnt over the years to deal with the presence of the unintegrated "gold consciousness" in his constitution and may take many years to get to the point of suicide.

Because the proving potence is a once-only situation (like taking a poison, or being exposed to an unusual bacteria) the immune/psychic system is at first overwhelmed. There is an extreme reaction in which extreme states of mind (like being suicidal) appear rapidly. This is analogous to the course of an acute disease or a poisoning. This is followed by the attempt to process and/or discharge the "invading" potence. The length of a proving is defined by the time it takes for the psyche/body to assimilate the presence of the proving potence. This is similar to an acute illness.

On the other hand the influences of life are chronic. They don't go away. In infancy our responses are acute. We laugh, cry and shriek in immediate response to life. Infants also get fevers from time to time. As self-consciousness develops we learn to avoid or deny the things that trouble us. In so doing we accumulate unresolved conflicts and problems. The acute action and reaction of infancy is gradually replaced by a more stable sense of self. However, this more stable sense of self can come at the expense of a stockpile of chronic problems.

In infancy there is little stable self-consciousness, and thus little residue of chronic problems (although there are of course inherited tendencies lying like seeds waiting to sprout in the soil of life's circumstances). The development of a stable sense of self leads, to one extent or another, to chronicity. It creates a need to cope and to keep troublesome thoughts, feelings and reactions under control. Thus acute episodes (of stress and response) can be replaced by more or less chronic patterns of ill health.

Ego and archetype

We encounter powers in heaven and earth greater than the human being; powers to which we are subject and which make life unpredictable; powers which we often seek to control. In the modern world it is assumed that we can control the powers of nature, be they germs or climatic conditions, if only we can acquire enough scientific knowledge.

It is also assumed that we can control the powers of nature within – archetypal drives and responses to life's eternal situations like mothering, fathering, homemaking, conflict, creativity, and so on – if only we can exert enough will power. In the past it was understood that the relationship with the powers of heaven and earth involved ritual and sacrifice. These powers were imagined as gods and goddesses with whom a harmonious relationship needed to be maintained. Through ritual, ancient peoples attempted to maintain the wholeness of nature and cosmos, which had been dangerously threatened by the emergence of human consciousness and activity.[12]

I am not, of course, recommending a return to a cosmos peopled by divinities of which we must live in superstitious fear. However I am saying that the human ego is a small power within the world of natural and psychological powers. We are easily overwhelmed by the forces of nature in their expression through disease agent, climate and other natural forces. We are equally likely to be overwhelmed by the powers within our own souls: love, hate, spirituality, sexuality, the situations of parenthood or childhood, of responsibility or dependence and many others. We can't control these inner demands, but we can learn to understand and co-operate with them. This needs understanding and imaginative dialogue with these deep and powerful domains within ourselves. To use the language of the ancient world, ritual and sacrifice are needed. We can't control nature, but we can learn to harmonise our activity with her ways and seasons.

The homœopathic way of knowledge

Now let's turn our attention to what might be termed a homœopathic "way of knowledge" that underpins homœopathic provings. Hahnemann suggests that participating in provings is the most direct and valid way of understanding the power to make sick and the power to heal that lies slumbering in a substance. He also saw provings as part of a way of self-knowledge.[13] In a proving the prover acquires direct experience of the powers of nature and the powers of their own psyche. In this respect homœopathy is a science and art rooted in direct experience of both outer and inner worlds.

In other words the homœopath is called upon, one way or another to have knowledge of the healing properties of nature (remedies), experience of the nature and forms of suffering, as well as knowledge of their own inner processes. The understanding of nature, the understanding of others and self-understanding all go hand in hand. A properly managed proving provides an opportunity to acquire more understanding of oneself, of the nature of disease and of the healing properties of natural things.

A proving evokes the mingling of the inner world of the soul and the outer world of nature. Thus the prover explores their psyche, not as an isolated entity, but as a part of nature. By this I mean that the prover explores their own inner world in its true context, not as an isolated entity, but as what it really is – a unique embodiment of the forces and elements of the world. Because we ourselves are made of the same elements and forces as the world and all that's in it, whatever enters from without will find its similarity within. Whatever note is sounded from without will arouse a similar resonance from within our own depths. As we have seen, individual constitution and the fabric of the world are one and the same. Thus the proving potence arouses the presence of that which is similar within. Snake will arouse snake, gold will arouse gold, and so on. If the inner "snake", or the inner "gold" has been repressed, or not yet encountered, then there will be difficulties to be faced during the proving.

Hahnemann suggested that provings were good for you.[14] They help you towards health. What can we make of a paradox in which what apparently poisons and disrupts your well-being could also be thought to be good for you? Putting aside puritanical notions of something that hurts being good for you, I would like to suggest that a prover is healthier after a proving because they have widened their perceptual framework. They have allowed something in that might normally be resisted. In this process something of what was unconscious has become conscious. In this sense the prover becomes a little freer from the burdens of unconscious responses. Their channels are thus, so to speak, more open. They have experienced more, had to face the previously unknown or unwanted, and either willingly or through necessity, have overcome some resistance.

In this sense, through the proving process, a prover becomes a more competent homœopath in "being" as well as knowledge. They live "like suffering" as well as knowing about it in theory.

Healing traditions and homœopathy

The approach to healing, and to becoming a healer, embodied in homœopathy is not essentially new. Rather it is part of a tradition that has always existed. It has been recognised since the earliest eras of human culture that the healer should know about healing properties of substances, understand the psychological or inner "spiritual" nature of disease, and should be wise in the ways of his own and other people's psyche.

The first healers that we know about were the shamans. For thousands of years shamanic healers was trained to have special knowledge of the spirit world as well as the medicinal power of plants.[15] We might say that shamans were the first experts in psychology and medicine. They were the early practitioners of a medicine for body and soul that exists in the world today in the form of homœopathy.

When considering provings in the light of this ancient tradition it is not surprising to find this description of the shaman's initiatory training:

"When the soul has reached maturity the bird carries it back to earth, cuts the candidate's body into bits, and distributes them among the evil spirits of disease and death. Each spirit devours the part of the body that is his share; this gives the future shaman power to cure the corresponding disease." [16]

Doesn't this sound, symbolically at least, a bit like the proving process we have been discussing? In a proving the prover surrenders to a power of nature. This power awakens corresponding powers within the psyche. While the proving lasts, the everyday world of the prover is broken up and disrupted. In this way the prover gains experiential insight into the spirits of nature and the "spirit powers" of the psyche. This makes the prover knowledgeable in the use of those remedies. A friend, an experienced prover, told me, "I now have twenty good remedies under my belt." She meant that she had first-hand experience of the nature and use of these remedies.

All of this requires a certain degree of maturity. I have seen that when provers enter into provings in a naive way, or when the proving is not well managed, disruption can be considerable. The life of the prover and those around them can be profoundly affected and in some cases severely disrupted. Provers can fall prey to overwhelming emotions and illusions.

The powers of nature are not to be messed about with, but should be approached with the kind of reverence that would have been considered essential for this kind of work by all traditional cultures.

When it comes to provings, the understanding that comes from familiarity with one's own nature and one's own inner processes is more than helpful. In fact I think there is an argument for some kind of inductive preparation for provers. I know that we don't want to prejudice the outcome of the proving in any way. However, if the prover at least has some kind of preparation for a journey into unknown realms then the fallout will be less and the experiences will be integrated more effectively, without reducing the value of the proving. After all, you wouldn't undertake a mountaineering trip without the proper equipment. It is a matter of record that most provings, from the time of Hahnemann to the present day, have in fact been undertaken by homœopaths, homœopathic students, as well as their friends and family. This suggests that the need for preparation has at least been intuited because such people, through contact with homœopathy, would in some degree be prepared for their experiences. When a person already familiar with the inner domain undertakes a proving, they will be better equipped to face and enter into the inner processes thus activated.

When the homœopath has journeyed in the realm of "spirit powers", has encountered the powers of nature as well as the archetypal powers of the psyche, then they are better prepared to undertake their healing work. They are ready "to return to earth."

Alchemy and homœopathy

The tradition of alchemy also sets a precedent for homœopathic work. Alchemy is believed to have originated in ancient Egypt. Via Islamic culture it formed an influential, though often hidden, body of knowledge right up to the age of enlightenment in Europe.[17] It was in decline in Hahnemann's day, but Hahnemann the scholar would almost certainly have been exposed to alchemical ideas and texts.[18]

Until Jung's serious psychological research into alchemy in the first half of the twentieth century, scholars had by and large dismissed alchemy as at worst nonsensical and at best the crude beginnings of chemistry. It had been regarded as the mumblings of deluded theorists who believed they could make gold from base metals. Jung stumbled upon alchemical texts and was struck by the similarity of the images that occur in the texts and the images that he had seen in the dreams and fantasies of his patients. This led Jung to research the previously dismissed texts. In essence what Jung said was; look, these texts are not talking literally, they are symbolic expressions of inner psychological processes. The true alchemists were in search of spiritual gold, not material gold.

Now, the curious thing about alchemical texts is that they abound with images and diagrams that are clearly partly chemical/scientific – pictures of distillation apparatus for example – and partly psychological in that they consist of the kind of archetypal imagery which Jung recognised as being characteristic of the collective unconscious. He maintained he had seen similar images arising spontaneously in the dreams of his patients and in the fantasies of psychotic patients. For this reason Jung believed that the explorations of the early alchemists, as well as forming the origins of chemistry, constituted early attempts towards what would later become his own formulations of depth psychology.

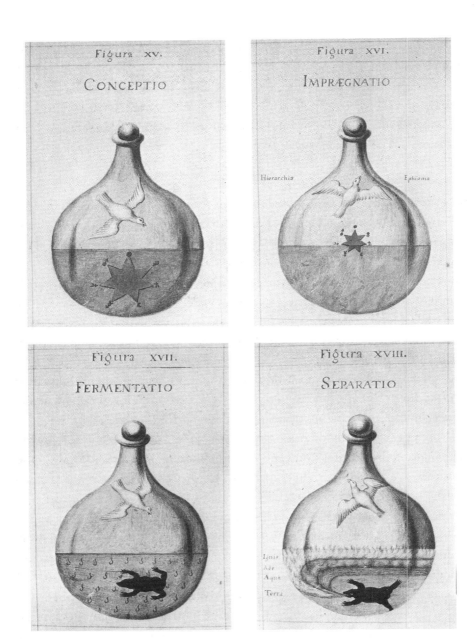

Fig. 11.1 Alchemical images

From a series of drawings, *Sapientia veterum philosophorum sive doctrina eorundem de summa et universali medicina*, 18th century, Bibliothèque de l'Arsenal, Paris, Ms. 974, fig. i-xxxvi, xxxixx, xl.

Jung believed that the images and psychological states experienced by these researchers were attributed by them to the chemical substances with which they experimented, only because, due to lack of knowledge of chemistry, they "projected" these experiences onto the chemical substances, incorrectly believing them to be the properties of these substances. Projection (where unconscious attributes of the observer are seen as properties of external events, people or objects) takes place in the darkness of the unknown. Jung surmised, no doubt at least partly correctly, that the scientific knowledge of a few centuries ago was indeed a "dark unknown" which invited these projections.[19]

While this may be partially true, homœopathic research shows that there is a connection between a given potentised substance and a corresponding psychological state which does not come about solely through projection. Thus when a substance is potentised, and the vibrational information is released, we encounter, in a proving, a meeting ground of an aspect of the spirit of nature and an aspect of the unconscious psyche of the individual. The prover explores the ground where the outer world of nature and the world of the human soul meet.

In a proving the field of the potence and the vital force of the prover interact and interpenetrate each other. The condition of the prover arises in response to the proving potence.

A proving response may even occur when the experimenter hasn't actually taken the potence. There is evidence to suggest that exposure to the field of a substance, without actually taking it, is enough to produce proving effects. For example it is not uncommon in group provings for those who haven't actually taken the "pill" to experience the alterations characteristic of the proving.[20] In the recent proving of Positronium some of the most powerful images, feelings and sensations were experienced by the chemist as she ran up the potency.[21] In other words the potence is a field that is experienced telepathically by sensitive individuals whether they take the pill or not.

We don't know if alchemical researchers actually took potences in the way that a prover does, although there is some evidence to suggest that they may have known about potentising procedures.[22] However, we can surmise that some alchemists at least contemplated their experiments carefully.

Is it too far fetched to suggest that the alchemist, through contemplation and meditation, through entering into the spirit of his experiments, was in some way subject to inner experiences that were evoked by, and arose from, the substance with which he was experimenting? As the alchemist experimented, proving-like experiences could have arisen. Perhaps this was through taking potences, or simply through the contemplation of the behaviour of substances in the laboratory. At any rate he or she (there were famous women alchemists) would also have been exposed to contact with toxic substances in the laboratory experiments, which would have produced poisoning effects in them.

The implications of the body of work left behind by the alchemists, and of the fact that psychological alterations are experienced in provings of potentised substances is far-reaching and as yet largely unresearched. It suggests that physical and psychological processes may be linked in as yet unsuspected ways.

There is already a growing body of scientific research to show that events in the mind and body are in fact woven into a single whole. This field of research, called psychoneuroimmunology (PNI), is demonstrating the effects of emotions, via the agency of nervous and immune systems, on physical health.[23]

Proving data goes further and hints at the possibility that the inner life of feeling, thought and imagination found in the human being is closely connected to the "inner life" of substance. In the making of a potency, the inner field or "idea" of a substance is freed from matter. When this potence is taken by the prover it awakens the aspects of the prover's inner life (images, feelings, sensations, thoughts) that correspond to the field of the potence.

A concluding thought

Is it possible, just as all matter is composed of the elements of the periodic table and that the functioning of the body can be explained in terms of biochemical compounds built up from those elements, that the inner psychic life of human beings is composed, in a way not yet recognised or understood, of the "inner life" of these same elements and compounds? If this were to be the case the implications would be far reaching. It would suggest that we are made of the world not only in the physical sense, but in the world of the imagination as well. It would be startling indeed if we were to discover that the stuff of the world were, in some sense as yet hardly dreamed of, living its inner life through the inner life of human beings in a similar way to which the material life of the elements of the periodic table comes to expression in the body of nature and human physical constitution.

Chapter 12:

Cure

In this chapter I want to take up the notion of cure. What does cure mean? Hahnemann suggests that cure is "the lifting of all the symptoms of the disease and of the entire complex of perceptible befallments." [1] At first glance this sounds a bit absolute and final. However, we might also think of Hahnemann's definition in more relative terms. From this perspective cure is a resolution of past wounds and difficulties – a resolution that allows one to live more fully in the present.

In the unfolding of individuality (Jung called this process "individuation"), wounds can be sustained at any stage. When this happens the subsequent stages in the differentiation of the self are hampered. Development then becomes one-sided. Difficulties arising from unresolved conflicts become buried. Thence dysfunctional patterns of a psychological or physical nature become part of the basis of a person's existence in the world. Psychological conflict is consigned to the shadow, forming the basis of repetitive and unconscious patterns of behaviour. The body steps in to carry the burden of dysfunction. All of this is further exacerbated by the presence of inherited or miasmatic traits.

Law of cure

Well-prescribed homœopathic remedies can help to reverse this process. They reach deep into psychological, cellular and ancestral history, bringing healing to body and soul. One of homœopathy's early pioneers, Constantine Hering, made important observations concerning the dynamics of cure.

Hering, famous among other things for a ten-volume materia medica and the first (involuntary!) proving of the notorious (though in actual fact not so dangerous) bushmaster snake (Lachesis muta muta),[2] was the first to formulate a homœopathic law of cure.[3] This law – Hering's law of cure – is really three laws in one. It states that during homœopathic treatment symptoms disappear from time present to time past, from within to without, and from above down.

The first requirement. Curative action reaches back into the patient's history.

Hering's first law states that symptoms disappear in the reverse order of appearance, implying that the action of remedy or remedies progresses from time present to time past, progressively unlocking and resolving the past.

An important additional observation, which is closely related to the first law, is that old symptoms can reappear during treatment. These are symptoms a person once had that apparently ceased to exist or were replaced by others. We have already seen that past difficulties become, as it were, out of sight but not out of mind. They slip below the horizons of consciousness becoming unconscious memories, latent patterns of functional disturbance in mind or body. Thus old symptoms and old memories are brought to the surface during the course of homœopathic treatment.

The second requirement. An integrative and harmonising function, older and more inclusive than individualised self -consciousness, is called upon.

Hering's second law says that cure takes place from within to without. At first sight this may seem at variance with what has just been said. In practise it means that the patient experiences a lightening of being and relaxation of tension as the first sign of the beneficial action of a remedy. It also means that lung symptoms, for example, will tend to get better before skin symptoms.

This activity suggests that, through the action of the remedy, a deep centre of being and wisdom within the patient is called upon. This centre has always been there, and always will be. It is older than the presence of human self-consciousness. It is the ground of being from which all arises, including our own consciousness, and into which all dies back. It is the ground that contains and includes wholeness as well as giving rise to all new growth and consciousness. Cure really means the reconnection with this eternal life-giving ground of being.

*The third requirement. A more embracing threshold of consciousness is estab-
lished.*

Hering's third law states that symptoms disappear from above down. This suggests that cure, in moving from above down, moves from the head as the seat of consciousness, to the body. In healing, what was denied or wounded (by self consciousness) needs to be understood and included (by consciousness).

Self-consciousness has its seat in the cerebral cortex. It is this conscious-ness that wounds. As consciousness emerges during the individual develop-mental process it can disrupt what existed before. For example the mental/conceptual self disrupts the unconscious symbiosis of the infant's emotional world. But differentiated self-consciousness has another important capacity. It can look back on the way it has come, see the damage that was caused, and set about healing old wounds. It can eventually look back at the traumas and wounds of infancy and childhood, and, from this higher and wider perspective, initiate healing practises. It is one of life's greatest paradoxes that conscious-ness is both that which wounds and agent of healing. From its differentiated perspective consciousness can acknowledge and describe the suffering of the whole.

In this sense healing must start from the perspective of self-conscious-ness (above) and spread downwards to embrace the wholeness of being.

Let's summarise these observations concerning the dynamics of cure:

Firstly, the curative process must be able to reach back into the past so that wounds that have been sustained can be healed and unresolved conflicts can be laid to rest.

Secondly, an integrative healing function must be called upon. This function is an activity of the ground out of which the self-conscious "I" emerges in the first place. This ground, which is able to hold and harmonise the totality of a person, as well as be the matrix that gives birth to the self conscious "I", is as the mother to the child.

Thirdly, the healing process must help a person to move on from old and unnecessary dysfunctions to a more embracing and inclusive way of being. In other words there must be movement towards a more embracing consciousness.

Disease, healing and consciousness

To help us in our attempt to understand what cure might entail I would like to return to Hahnemann's theory of psora. Through his researches Hahnemann arrived at the conclusion that one primal disease lay at the root of the myriad forms of suffering that afflict humankind. Hahnemann called this primal disorder psora, which means "the itch". According to him the itch disease lies slumbering in the depths of human constitution and is roused into activity by adverse circumstances of life.

He noted that the primary manifestation of this disease is a highly contagious acute infection that produces a terrible itching of the skin.[4] The sufferer is driven to relentless scratching, but this does not relieve. In Hahnemann's day this "itch diathesis" was sometimes known as scabies. (In Hahnemann's day however the term scabies covered many other affections besides the one now known as scabies).[5] Hahnemann also maintained that the itch disease had previously appeared as a form of leprosy (descriptions dating from about 3500 years ago are recorded in the bible), characterised by an inveterate and violent itching.[6] Hahnemann held that the various forms of chronic disease of mind and body come into being as the result of the suppression of the primary manifestation, the itching skin eruption, of psora.[7]

Also implicit in Hahnemann's writings is the idea that man was susceptible to the contagious itch disease (scabies, etc.) because of a deeper latent disease, a disease that lay at the very core of man's being.[8] Kent was more explicit, both about susceptibility and the nature of the deeper disease. Kent states that man is susceptible to disease because of derangements in thinking and willing. In other words (as I suggested in Chapter 7) the origins of disease lie in the perceptions and consequent activities of self-consciousness.[9]

What can we make of these assertions? Do they make any sense in respect of what has been said so far about consciousness, disease and healing? Let's inquire a little further.

I have suggested that chronic disease is fundamentally a problem of consciousness. Hahnemann proposes that psora is the root cause of chronic disease. Do these two propositions support each other?

The primary manifestation of psora, according to Hahnemann, is an itching of the skin which, in its most unbridled form, no amount of scratching will relieve. Could there be a link between the itch disease of the skin and the problems consequent to the emergence of self-consciousness? Let's turn to embryology to see if there is any basis for the possible relationship between the itch of the skin and the suffering brought about by consciousness.

Embryology tells us that the ectoderm in the human embryo gives rise to the epidermis of the skin and epithelium of skin glands. It also gives rise to the tissues of the nervous system including the central and peripheral systems. In other words there is an early structural relationship between the outer layer of the skin on the one hand, and the nervous system on the other. Let's look at this structural connection a little further.

Skin

The skin is the outer border of the body. It's where your physical body ends and the environment begins. It is now known that the skin is a biochemically highly complex and sensitive organ, rich in nerve endings and their associated cells.[10] Thus in a certain sense we can think of the skin as a part of the nervous system. It is an omnidirectional sense organ, facilitating the most fundamental and undifferentiated experience of the world. The skin mediates, at a fundamental level, between what's outside and what's inside.

Touch is a crucial sense through which the infant first establishes its relationship with the environment. It is in the very early stages of infant development that the sense of physical presence in relationship to the world is formed (see Chapter 3). The first stage in the development of a sense of self comes about through the way the infant touches the world, and is touched by the world (most especially the mother).

Nervous system

Through the skin and associated senses, the first sense of a differentiated self emerges. (Orifices, like the nose, mouth or anus, are the places where the skin folds into the body to become an internalised skin. The epithelium of mouth and nose are formed from the ectoderm, as are the sensory epithelial of nose and ear structures, as well as the lens of the eye and the retina. We can see then that in a certain sense the specialised senses are at once specialised epidermis and specialised nervous apparatus. The skin and specialised sense organs together make up the organ of touch. The world "touches" you not only through your skin, but also through sight, hearing, smell and taste.)

The skin and associated senses thus mediate between the primal self and the world. The nervous system is also a mediator. The sympathetic nervous system helps maintain balanced functioning in the internal systems of the body. The central nervous system is more particularly involved in receiving stimuli and impressions from the external world. It also mediates the activities – including the higher functions of consciousness – which arise in response to this input.

The brain itself has an inner and outer structure. It has an outer surface as well as inner, deeper structures. The deeper structures are far older than the surface structures and are concerned with our most primitive and instinctual responses.

In the 1960's, American researcher Paul MacLean put forward the notion of a triune brain.[11] He suggested that the brain could actually be conceived of as three brains in one. He called these the reptilian, paleomammalian and neomammalian brains.

The reptilian brain is located on the brain stem, an upward growth of the spinal cord. It is the most primitive part of the brain, shared with all other vertebrates. This brain is concerned purely with the maintenance of life, instinct and survival. Its behaviour is determined by instinctual precedent.

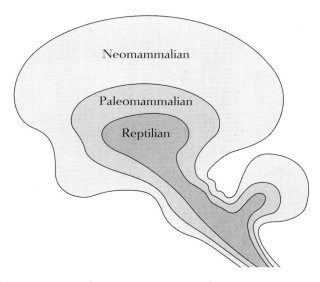

Fig. 12.1 Triune Brain (after MacLean, 1973)

The paleomammalian brain comprises the mid brain and limbic system. It includes a primitive cortex, which gives lower animals greater ability to adapt to the internal and external environment. The limbic system (including hippocampus, hypothalamus, thalamus) balances and controls instincts and hormone levels. The paleomammalian brain is related to self preservation and preservation of the species, and is concerned especially with fundamental emotions like fear, anger, and sexual attraction.

The neomammalian brain is synonymous with the neocortex, the two hemispheres that dominate (literally and symbolically!) the brains of higher mammals. The neocortex receives its information largely from the external environment. It is externally orientated and is concerned with cognition and sophisticated perceptual processes as opposed to instinctive and affective behaviour.[12]

In short then the older structures controlling primitive instinctual responses and activities and primal emotional responses lie within and below. The structures that facilitate the higher functions of the nervous system lie on the outside and above. MacLean refers to these three brains as the reptilian (the oldest), the paleomammalian and the neomammalian (the newest).

The cerebral cortex is the outer layer of the cerebrum. It is associated with sensory perception via touch and the specialised senses, as well as the initiation of voluntary muscle control and action. In it are found the higher centres associated with memory, thinking, reasoning, and so on.

The cerebral cortex then is the upper and outer surface of the brain, which facilitates the conscious activity which constitutes, so to speak, the upper and outer surface of the human psyche. This consciousness is, as Jung has shown, the surface of an enormous depth of psyche. In evolutionary terms this kind of discriminative consciousness is relatively recent. It mediates between the reality of the outer world and the primal drives, responses and emotions of the primitive subconscious psyche located in the lower centres of the paleomammalian and reptilian brains. Thus the activity (conscious discrimination), which constitutes the surface of the enormous and ancient depth of psyche, takes place in the surface structure that covers a far older brain.

Structural and functional correspondences

I'd like to take this analogy a step further. There is, I suggest, a structural and functional correspondence between the skin as the surface of the body, the cerebral cortex as the surface of the brain, and human self-consciousness as the surface of the ancient and deep collective unconscious. Thus, activity in one area – according to the laws of correspondence – would be reflected in activity in another.

In human evolution, self-consciousness differentiates out of the older evolutionary matrix of nature. As this evolutionary developmental activity is replayed, in microcosm, in the emergence of individual self-consciousness through infancy and beyond, conflict arising from this process – conflict between sense of self and the demands/expectations of the world – would show up in the very place, the very boundary, at which this sense of a separate self is first formed. In short, primary conflict arising from the meeting of consciousness of self (seated in the cerebral cortex) and the world, would appear on the outer perimeter of the nervous system, namely the epidermis of the skin.[13]

Is there any evidence to support this developmental view of psora? Atopic eczema, a sensitive reactivity of the skin, although not infectious, is a typical expression of the itch disease. It is often associated with a family history of eczema and asthma. It is otherwise known as infantile eczema because it typically appears in infants around three or four months old.[14] It is at about this age, research has suggested, that physical self-consciousness first starts to differentiate.[15] The infant, at around this age, starts to realise that its physical body is different from the physical environment. In other words the first stage of the differentiation of the self is underway. The first steps on the path of individuation are being taken. Is it surprising then that the first signs of separation anxiety should reveal itself at about this time? If this is the case then it would of course be expressed somatically (as an itch of the skin that expresses the anxiety of self consciousness), as there is as yet no conceptual self to attempt to articulate the problem.

The skin and wholeness

The skin is an omnidirectional sense organ. It thus mediates an experience of the world as an undivided whole. Spiritual psychologist, Robert Sardello, puts it well:

"The organ for sensing the world as a synthesis of the whole, for sensing particularities and yet at the same time sensing that everything is indeed related to everything else, is the skin ... The body experiences the surrounding world as a whole through a sensing that is like touch, but this sensing through touch does not necessarily involve being physically touched. The body knows its surroundings through touch, which also occurs from a distance, in principle, any distance. While the skin is the organ for experiencing the touch of the world, it does not have to be in physical contact with what touches it any more than the eye has to be in physical contact with an object in order to see it. Through practising attentiveness to the body, the sense of touch can become a conscious way of experiencing the world, not as a world of objects, but as a world of activity." [16]

The sense of individual self first emerges through the mediation of skin and nervous system. This primal self experiences itself and the world not as sharply differentiated, but as the wholeness of itself and the wholeness of the world as an intimate and interrelated whole.

However it often happens in the course of development that there is disappointment or trauma. This teaches the self to withdraw behind the boundaries of the skin. Thus the self becomes progressively convinced that it is a separate self that must struggle for survival. The flow of exchange between inner and outer which first gives rise to a sense of self is ruptured. The self now becomes an isolated "thing" (rather than a dynamic process), preoccupied with defence and survival.

The skin can be the mediator of unity and exchange with the world. It can also become an irritating – and irritated – reminder of the self's separation from the world.

The oldest disease

We have looked at psora in terms of the origins of the appearance of individual consciousness in infancy. What about psora as a concomitant to the appearance of an individualised self-consciousness in the evolution of man? This is a large and complex subject that we can only touch on here. Hahnemann maintained that the "itch disease" is the primitive disease of mankind, appearing in different forms in different historical periods (scabies in his day and leprosy at the dawn of written records). According to him it is older than the oldest history of the oldest race.[17] In other words psora points to an ancient disruption of human wholeness. This suggests then that psora points to the origins of consciousness in human evolution, just as it points to the origins of self-consciousness in the life of the infant.

Comparative mythologists see the history of the evolution of consciousness told in the great myths of the world. It is the story of the temptation by the serpent and the expulsion from the garden. It is the story of the theft of fire by Prometheus, the champion of human kind, in the face of the wrath of Zeus. In these great mythological stories the hero, the symbol of human self-consciousness, undergoes a traumatic birth, has to struggle to overcome archetypal powers, and finally finds his way home, finds the treasure or finds wholeness in a sacred marriage. The outcome of these stories symbolises the way in which self-consciousness, having become aware of its self as separate and thus become self-responsible, has to seek a new union with the holy matrix from which it was born. In doing this it brings the gifts of consciousness to the service of life.

Chapter 13:

Some notes on case taking and case analysis

The purpose of the homœopathic interview is to arrive at an understanding of the patient as a whole. On this basis the remedy that most closely matches the patient may be given.

Symptom and context

The homœopath is guided to this remedy through matching definite symptoms in the patient's case to the known symptoms of a remedy.

Definitive symptoms, however, are not isolated entities existing in a vacuum. They exist in a context. They are like the individual brush strokes that exist against a background on the painter's canvas. It is this background or context that gives symptoms meaning and value, and enables the homœopath to recognise individual symptoms as part of a characteristic whole.

By "context" I mean all overall perceptions, classifications and structures that aid in the perception of the patient as a whole. These include notions such as essence[1] and central delusion.[2] Also included is analysis by kingdom, periodic table, and plant or animal family. In the notion of context I also include all maps such as those of the elements (mappa mundi) and miasms (Hahnemann, Ortega, Sankaran, etc.).

In "context" we may also include notions of signature or symbol, in as much as these might be suggestive of particular remedies. By "signature" I mean what is known of the form, composition, function and behaviour of a particular mineral, plant or animal. By "symbol" I mean the complex of meanings and associations that have arisen in different cultures in connection with a particular mineral, plant or animal.

In this view of case data, specific symptoms are foreground and context is background. Context gives meaning and value to specific symptoms. On the other hand if we put context in the foreground and ignore or downgrade definitive symptoms we are far more likely to go astray. More of this later in the chapter.

Symptoms

The patient may come with presenting symptoms, concomitant symptoms and/or chronic symptoms. They may also report symptoms that they had in the past. The symptoms may be general or local. They may pertain to mind or body.

Within all this complexity we are looking for the pattern that connects. We are looking for the activity of the dynamis. This may be apparent in someone's thoughts, imagination, feelings or sensations. It may be in sensation, action or modality.

It is not so important whether the symptoms pertain to thought, imagination, emotion or physical function. However, it is important to choose symptoms that express an individual's fundamental experience and/or his reactions to this experience. For example, as we saw in Chapter 6, pressure could be a fundamental perception and loosening a fundamental (re)action. For another individual the desire to perform may be central. It's what she does or desires to do (action). We can ask, "what lies behind this need?" A need to be admired. What lies within the need to be admired? The feeling or perception of not being admired. What lies within this? A feeling of being a failure. This feeling is painful, thus defended, and therefore harder to see. What we actually see is achievement and performance.

Guiding symptoms may be found in the patient's presenting complaint, in concomitant symptoms, in chronic symptoms, and sometimes as a symptom from the past. Wherever they come from these symptoms should express something about a person's perceptions, their actions or reactions, as well as modalities.

We have to ask ourselves, in what way is the subconscious domain of the vital force expressing itself? We take note of deep-rooted beliefs, of what someone imagines to be so, of images, feelings and emotions, and of sensations. The further away from consciousness, the better. The more outside the domain of rationality, the better. For example, stitching pain in the eye is more characteristic as a symptom than a feeling of disappointment. The former is a striking and uncontrived expression of the vital force. The latter is a typical (and thus not unusual or striking) human response (i.e. mental interpretation of a situation) to not getting what one had hoped for. On the other hand fear of sharp things (Spigelia anthelmia) concomitant to stitching pains in the eye is striking. The fear here echoes the vital sensation.

Having noted the sensations, feelings, images or beliefs, we note the actions and reactions connected with these perceptions. We also note the modalities. Any or all of this data, if it is striking or characteristic, can lead to the similimum.

Selection of symptoms

When the homœopath needs to select a symptom, or symptoms, that best reflect the nature of the case, three questions will help to clarify what's valuable and what isn't.

The three questions are:

• how high/deep?
• how striking/unusual?
• how true/reliable?

Let's look at these three.

How high/deep?

The patient may reveal deeply rooted beliefs and feelings. The patient's dreams may be indicative of her innermost state. Through such symptoms we glimpse her inner landscape. However, these kinds of expression are often difficult to match to a particular remedy with any degree of certainty. It is often better to go with more reliable symptoms and then see if the remedy arrived at could match (on the basis of the descriptions found in the materia medicas) the feelings and delusions of the patient (see below). Reliable symptoms are generally found amongst the clearly defined and striking generals, physicals, mentals or modalities. Sensations are important if striking. Actions and reactions are also of great value, as are modalities, desires and aversions.

How striking/unusual?

This asks how characteristic of the patient is the symptom. How expressive of the pattern of disturbance in the patient is the symptom? The striking can appear in any guise on any level. The striking can reveal itself in the language of the patient, in dreams or in any marked psychological or general characteristic. It can reveal itself in the physical particulars and sensations. The symptom may be striking because unusual, or striking because of its intensity. It may be striking through being symbolic of the patient's inner life.

Thus the psyche or dynamis may show itself in any striking symptom. From this point of view the whole repertory becomes a repertory of the psyche. We may find the characteristic symptom that expresses the inner nature of the patient in any section of the repertory.

How true/reliable?

How sure am I that this bit of data is actually there, and I didn't make it up or project it? Something that scores highly with the other two questions might not score well here. For example a patient dreams that an animal is being killed. This dream scores well on the first question, how deep or high? It is an expression of the unconscious psyche of the patient and is thus a message from the inner reaches of the patient's psyche. It scores well on the second question, how striking? It is very striking in that it reveals a condition of the patient in which some aspect of her instinctual life is suffering. It expresses the essential condition of the patient.

But can I use this data to base a prescription on? Could I repertorise such symptoms? I might look at rubrics that express the theme of killing, or rubrics to express the theme of animals. Would such rubrics be a correct interpretation of the case data? Maybe and maybe not. It might be that the required remedy is in one of these rubrics. On the other hand it might not. Rubrics that directly express the inner life of the patient (such as dreams and delusions) are often under represented, misrepresented, or just plain misleading.

On the other hand we can be fairly sure of the veracity of physical sensations and dysfunctions. Cramping is cramping. A green discharge is a green discharge. But when it comes to the mind there are many overlaps and ambiguities of meaning. Different provers or different clinical observers could have expressed the same thing in different words. For example can we be sure of the difference between "anxiety of conscience", "delusion, has done wrong", "delusion, has committed a crime", and "delusion, is a criminal". At the very least there is an ambiguity of meaning. We might choose one of these rubrics, when in fact the required remedy appears in one of the other rubrics. So cramping in the calves may be more reliable as a guiding symptom (especially when we see that the patient experiences their whole being as "cramped") than the feeling of having done wrong. We need to be careful not to pin things down too much. We need to keep a flexibility of approach.

As we've seen, specific symptoms appear against a contextual background that gives them meaning and pattern. Context refers to descriptions of essence or central delusion; analysis by kingdom, periodic table, plant family, animal group, and so on; consideration of miasms, elements etc.; also signature, symbolic understanding, and so on. Sometimes we are guided by specific symptoms and sometimes by context. The homœopath feels most confident when symptoms and context give a unified picture. This is the ideal for every case. We often, however, have to rely either more on specific symptoms or more on an understanding of context.

It is easy to make the mistake of giving too much value to context and not enough to the individual symptoms. Conversely we can overvalue individual symptoms and lose sight of the nature of the whole. An imbalance in either direction will not produce deep-acting results.

The final say in a homœopathic prescription should arise out of the artistic knowing which gathers up the separate facts into a wholeness that seems and feels right.

Intuition works the basic facts into a meaningful whole. One can nourish the intuitive function through study – study of human nature, the nature of sickness, remedy pictures, nature herself (plants, animals, etc.), symbolism and myth. All these strands enlarge our capacity to understand and open up channels of intuitive understanding. Through study we lay down more stepping-stones into further reaches of understanding. It helps us to access the collective unconscious. It helps us to plug in to the pool of wisdom and knowledge, which goes beyond the limitations of a personal psyche.

The repertory

It is important to remember that the repertory is an index and guide, and not the final arbiter. It is a listing, like a dictionary. A dictionary seeks to define specific words. To do this it treats the words as isolated entities. However to really understand words we must hear them and see them in the context of spoken or written language.

The same applies to symptoms in the repertory. They have been isolated from their context of whole experiences undergone by provers or patients. These whole experiences have been broken down into component parts called symptoms. In this process the wholeness of the original experience is lost. We now have a list of components (symptoms).

As a guide the repertory should be used with the right balance of discipline and imagination. The aim is that in matching the components (separate symptoms) to the components listed in the repertory, we will be led back to the wholeness of the case, now in possession of the similimum.

One might call this the way of analysis. Used with skill and imagination it can get us to the desired goal. Sometimes, when we know the remedy well, we can bypass this process altogether. We see the wholeness of the patient's state and know from previous experience of other patients the remedy that matches the state.

It's also possible that we've had direct experience of the remedy ourselves. Hahnemann's vision was that homœopaths should prove remedies on themselves.[3] In this way, through direct experience of the remedy state, the homœopath can recognise the same state in another. Hahnemann's "shamanic" vision, that the homœopath should be a living repository of materia medica, is only realisable to a limited extent. In most cases it is not possible for homœopaths to prove large numbers of remedies on themselves. This being the case the method of repertorial analysis became central to homœopathy.

In spite of this, as we've seen, it is still possible to go beyond analysis, and to enter with the patient into a more direct experience of their inner state. With courage we can help them to become aware of their thoughts, feelings and sensations as they actually are. This move beyond the boundaries of rationality and logical explanation can lead to a clearer perception of the patient's state. We then attempt to match this to a similar state produced by a remedial substance. To do this we need to continually deepen our understanding of remedy states through participation in provings, and where that isn't possible, through contemplation of published provings as well as study of the symptoms, nature, signature and symbolism of remedies and remedy groups.

Case taking
The Hahnemannian method
Hahnemann directs that the homœopath should simply let the patient describe their condition in their own words. Direct questioning should be kept to a minimum, mainly reserved for clarifying the nature of symptoms. He points out that unnecessary questioning can prevent the natural and spontaneous expression of the patient, thus distorting the picture described.[4]

This form of case taking is essentially passive. The patient is encouraged to talk with a minimum of interference. It requires that the homœopath should cultivate the posture of an empty vessel. As my first teacher used to say, "look, listen and don't think". I still find this sound advice. This emptiness creates the conditions and the space in which the patient's story can unfold.

Ambience and receptivity are of the greatest importance. The patient may talk about painful and long defended issues. Realisations and insights may be made. If there are silences, these should in general be allowed. If after a short while the patient seems to have nothing more to say, a gentle nudging along will be helpful. Open-ended prompts are the most useful: "How was that?" "How does that feel?" "Tell me more about that?" "What was that like?"

Some of the information given by the patient may be incomplete. It may be necessary to clarify the nature of a sensation, or a locality, or a modality. However, leading questions get misleading answers. General questions, such as, "Does weather or climate affect you at all?" are much better than "do thunderstorms effect you?" To this latter question the patient is almost bound to say yes, thus possibly giving a misleading answer. Almost everyone has a response of some kind to thunderstorms! What we are interested in is whether the person has a marked or outstanding reaction to them.

The active approach

To gain a deep understanding of the unconscious dynamics of a patient the Hahnemannian approach is sometimes inadequate on its own. We sometimes need to inquire further or follow a line of questioning. Of course, this needs to be done with sensitivity and respect for the patient's boundaries.

In both approaches the aim is to go beyond surface understanding. In the active approach this is done by following the line of the patient's expressions until the unconscious condition behind the expressions is more clearly revealed. In this method the homœopath comes back to open questions and prompts like "how does that feel?" and "tell me more?" and so on, until the underlying state of the patient becomes clearer. In this approach it is even more important that questions remain general and open prompts. The homœopath avoids introducing any of his or her own words or notions. If words are used they should be those of the patient. For example if the patient says "I feel constricted in the chest", the homœopath might, after a suitable pause, say, "constricted in the chest?" thereby inviting the patient to enter a little deeper into the feeling or the sensation.

Deep down we all carry certain feelings and sensations. These are often more or less chronic. These feelings and sensations are areas of vulnerability and sensitivity. Thus they are defended and unconscious.

Often a patient can tell you quite easily about what they do in life – their habits and reactions – but not so easily about their underlying feelings. For example if a person carries a deep feeling of hurt, in response to which they are always busy, they will probably be more aware of the busyness than the hurt. When you say to them, "How does it feel?" they are likely to say, "Oh, I just keep busy." In other words they jump to the action (busyness) and avoid the feeling (hurt). This is because the hurt is a place of vulnerability. It is buried or defended.

A further important point here is that "hurt" is just a word. It's a box or concept, which contains a feeling or complex of feelings. By using the label "hurt" we often keep the actual experience of the feeling at a distance. The word says little of the actual feeling or sensation that may be encapsulated within it. We may want to find out more about what lies within that word "hurt." To do this we may need to gently hold the patient in the place of hurt so that they can describe the actual feeling buried within the word. At this point the mind may try to go into concepts and explanations, or a description of what they do (keep busy, eat, avoid company, etc.) when this feeling is around. However it is also at this point that the patient may be able to go deeper. In response to further prompts like, "Can you describe hurt?" he or she might say things like, "Boiling in the chest", "My world is collapsing", "I'm alone and hated", and so on. We have gone beyond a concept (hurt) to an actual feeling or sensation.[5]

If it's necessary, in order to clarify understanding, to go a little deeper, different paths may be followed. For example how did they feel in such and such a situation? How does the presenting complaint make them feel? (In other words what is the underlying feeling or sensation in the presenting complaint?) How do they feel in situations of stress? What were their feelings as a child? By following one or any of these lines and by using each description of feeling or sensation as a stepping-stone to go a bit further into the underlying state, the patient's basic feelings and attitudes are revealed. One can also switch from one line of inquiry like how do you feel under stress, to another, such as how did you feel as a child? Or the patient may spontaneously jump from one line to another. With gentle and careful encouragement one can take the patient beyond their habitual actions into their underlying feelings or sensations. As this inner domain is revealed it becomes more obvious how feelings, actions, physical symptoms and life situations revolve around a single locus. This takes us a step closer to the deep acting similimum.

From outside to inside

The "outside" of the patient – the external manifestation of the human holon – is observable in symptom, alteration of function, behaviour, gesture, body language, facial expression, and so on. To build a symptom picture from such data is often quite adequate, especially in the hands of a good prescriber. However, to get good results from deep-acting remedies this method is dependent on the homœopath's capacity to choose just those symptoms that best manifest or symbolise the inner condition of the patient. Correct choice of symptoms leads to a deep-acting remedy. Incorrect choice of symptoms leads to a more superficial remedy.

To have more certainty about your prescription it may be necessary to go beyond the external manifestation of symptom, dysfunction, locality and observable behaviour. It may also be necessary because of a lack of manifest symptoms. It then becomes necessary to journey with the patient into their inner domain using the techniques described above.

When you do this you go beyond the rational consciousness of the patient. You go beyond the part that justifies, excuses and has a reason for everything. You journey beyond the boundaries of logic and rational description. You enter the domain of the unconscious. This is the world of irrational beliefs, images, feelings and sensations (see Chapter 6). At this deeper level one can often perceive the relationship between thoughts, feelings, sensations and actions (and sometimes life situations as well). We have a better chance of understanding the case as a single whole, and thus a better chance of finding the right remedy for the patient.[6]

A unified map

Hahnemann and the physician philosophers who followed him instruct that we should be led by guiding symptoms. These are symptoms that stand out as being indicative of the patient's inner dynamics.

We have also established that symptoms are seen in context. It is context that gives value and significance to symptoms. Ideas of essence, central delusion, kingdom, miasm, and so on, give context to specific symptoms.

During the case taking and analysis procedure we might bear in mind the following.

Kingdoms

From which kingdom is the required remedy?

If a mineral remedy, from which series of the periodic table? Given a possible series, is it in the early, middle or late phases of that series? In other words which vertical column does the remedy belong to? It is important to remember that salts have themes of more than one series and more than one vertical column. For example Kali carbonicum has the theme of series four, stage one (Kali) and series two, stage ten (carbon). From this point of view it is important to know the chemical composition of a substance.

If a plant, to which plant family does the remedy belong? Here it is necessary to know the common themes that run through a plant family. Leading homœopaths such as Rajan Sankaran, Jan Scholten and Massimo Mangialavori have been researching this area for some years. According to Sankaran it is a common sensation that unites the different species of a plant family. For example the common sensations of the Anacardiaceae family, which includes Rhus toxicodendron and Anacardium orientale, are "caught, stiff, tension, stuck, cramps, pressing." [7]

If an animal remedy, to which animal group does it belong? Here we may be guided by a striking symptom such as the desire for oranges or extreme sensitivity to noise of Theridion (Latrodectus curacaviensis, the orange spider). However, guiding symptoms will often point to an animal family as much as to a particular species. For example the well-known Lachesis symptom of sensitivity to clothing around the neck is a marked symptom of snakes in general. In fact, although it is a symptom particularly striking in snakes, it is also marked in animal remedies in general (Apis, Lac canninum, Sepia, etc.). From this we may suppose that the sense of constriction caused by clothing around the neck is indicative of the split between body and mind, or instinct and control, which is characteristic of animal remedies in general.

Miasms

Miasms can be important. The miasm indicates a person's basic stance in life. For example a person can be hopeful (psora), fixed and rigid (sycosis) or desperate (syphilis). Or they may be at another point along the spectrum of possibilities (see Chapter 7).

With mineral remedies, as we have seen, it helps to know which stage of a series of the periodic table that a person is in (stages 1 - 18). The periodic table can help us to see which phase of the life cycle a person is in. Are they stuck in the mode of beginnings, establishment or decline? Because plants and animals aren't in the periodic table we need other maps to help us perceive underlying themes in a case. The miasm map offers a similar idea of ascent, peak and decline. Sankaran's ten-miasm map helps us to see if the patient is struggling (ascent), accepting (peak), or trying to hold on (decline).

When the ten miasms are looked at as points on a cycle they fall into the pattern of beginning, middle and end (subdivided into ten phases – acute at the beginning, syphilis at the end). In his map each miasm expresses a different mode of reaction and coping.[8]

When a person is in the acute miasm, feelings and reactions are sudden and overwhelming. This is somewhat like the position of the infant who just feels and reacts in the moment, who has no forethought or analysis. Thus the acute miasm is the posture of someone at the beginning of life (like stage 1 in the periodic table). Remedies such as Aconite and Belladonna belong to the acute miasm.

The psoric feels faced by a challenge, which, with effort, can be overcome.

The sycotic miasm represents the position of the person established in life (or a life situation such as a relationship or job). Everything they feel and do is marked by a fixed posture in which they attempt to maintain the established status quo, whatever that happens to be. In order to do this they must hide aspects of themselves that don't fit with this established position. Thus the sycotic miasm represents the middle of life. It is a fixed place where one hides weaknesses. Thuja is a typical sycotic remedy. If a person reacts and copes in an acute manner, then the remedy will not be Thuja, even if specific symptoms suggest Thuja.

The cancer miasm comes between sycosis and syphilis. The person desperately (syphilis) tries to keep control (sycosis) of a situation where it is already beyond their capacity to impose order. Life is seen as a disintegrating situation – like cancer itself. This is the posture of someone for whom life, or a life situation, is in decline, or is at least imagined to be in decline. A striving for control, order and perfection is indicative of the cancer miasm. The posture of one in the syphilitic miasm is despairing and destructive. It is a hopeless situation. It is the end. The other miasms lie at intervals along the spectrum from acute to syphilitic – typhoid between acute and psoric, malaria between acute and sycosis, ringworm between psora and sycosis, tubercular between sycosis and syphilis, leprosy going towards syphilis. (See Chapter 7)

Miasms, plants and animals

An understanding of the miasmatic map helps to differentiate between one remedy and another. The map helps one to place the underlying drives and perceptions in a patient. The basic framework in the patient should match the basic framework of the remedy. (Thuja is not an acute remedy, and thus is not indicated in a patient with an acute posture, even if specific symptoms suggest it).

Sankaran has suggested that this map is particularly helpful when it comes to differentiating between plant remedies from the same botanical family. His clinical findings suggest that while different remedies from one family can have widely differing symptoms, they have underlying "themes" in common. For him this basic theme takes the form of a sensation. In other words different plants from one family, whilst being different in many respects, share common sensations.[9]

Understanding the miasm gives you a better chance of selecting the correct remedy from the plant family. For example if the patient has the posture of the cancer miasm (perfectionism, control, etc.), then the remedy must also reflect this posture. Thus, for example, someone needing Anacardium orientale relates to the sense of being caught or stuck (Anacardiaceae family) through the mode of the cancer miasm – through perfectionism and control. The rubrics are:

- Rest; cannot, when things are not in proper place (i.e. must have order)
- Delusions, imaginations; superhuman; control, is under (the superhuman power is part of their own makeup, driving them to superhuman achievement)

Animals also belong to miasmatic groups. For example, Theridion (and spiders in general) belongs to the tubercular miasm.[10] However, it is generally easier to see specific animal qualities in a person than specific plant qualities. Therefore a map such as the miasmatic map may not be as necessary for animals.

Miasms as doorways

We saw in Chapter 7 that miasms represent phases in the natural cycle of events. Thus miasms are like thresholds or doorways in the eternal cycle of birth and death. Each miasm represents a place in that cycle. Each miasm is a station in this process.

Each station, each doorway, asks that we leave something behind and enter something new. To do this successfully we must loosen our identity with what went before, so that we can embrace what is to come. The doorway becomes a place of sickness – a miasm – if we become stuck at that place. If we identify with beginnings we are always at the beginning. If we identify with holding an established position, we might always be fixed and rigid. If we identify with endings we could often be despairing, approaching life events with an attitude of despair.

Miasm	Sick mode	Healthy mode
Acute	Panic.	Alertness and reactivity.
Typhoid	Losing position of comfort. Intense short effort.	Alertness and survival.
Psora	Failure. Lack of confidence.	Meeting the challenge. Persistence.
Malaria	Stuck and intermittently attacked. Persecuted. Unfortunate.	Fight for independence. Stand up for rights.
Ringworm	Alternation between struggle and resignation.	Not giving up.
Sycosis	Cover up of fixed weakness.	Acceptance, of limits, of self, of the situation. Beginning of self-knowledge.
Cancer	Chaos and need to control.	Acceptance of chaos and breakdown as the matrix of new birth.
Tubercular	Suffocation. Suppressed. Compressed. No air. Need to get out.	Reaching beyond the material to the world of spirit.
Leprosy	Isolated. Despised.	No longer defined by the group. True to yourself.
Syphilis	Despair. Destruction.	Letting go of attachment. Death and rebirth.

Fig. 13.1 The ten miasms. Suggested sick and healthy modes.

Thus the miasm is a place of potential and possibility. It can also be a root of sickness. The miasm itself is neutral – simply a threshold in the order of things. When we become identified with that threshold we are held in its grip until we find a way forward.

We understand each miasm as a pattern of sickness. However, we can also view each miasm as the failure or distortion of a particular quality or attribute. I've given a schema of Sankaran's ten miasms, listed with their "pathological" characteristics as well as (suggested) positive qualities (Fig. 13.1).

This view of the miasms echoes the map of the development of consciousness presented in Chapter 3. It pictures thresholds on the path from infancy to old age. We may also see it as the journey from the embryonic self-consciousness of the infant, to the self-transcending consciousness of the sage.

This miasmatic map also pictures the cycle of any undertaking – be it a life, a relationship, an idea – from its inception, through its establishment, decline and death. However, it also suggests ways in which we might transcend the inevitability of this cycle. We don't have to remain identified with the "material" of something. In other words we can be in something – a life, a relationship, a profession, even an idea – but not wholly possessed by it. We can be spiritually free and independent while giving our all to what we are called to do.

Towards a developmental map for all kingdoms

The periods of the periodic table, as we have seen, correspond to the stages in the development in self-consciousness. It may also be possible to relate the pathology of plant and animal remedies to these developmental stages.

In fact Dr. Rupal Desai has already suggested a schema in which plant families correspond to basic human issues. This is her schema:

1a. Dependence (for survival) and procreation. (Fungi)
1b. Survival and growth despite strong adversities. (Coniferae)
1c. Dependent plus instinctual. (Apocynaceae, Scrophularaceae)
2. Strong instincts. (Solanaceae, Rutaceae, Piperaceae)
3. Emotions. (Cannabinaceae, Loganiaceae, Euphorbiaceae, Umbelliferae, Malvaceae)
4. Identity. (Compositae, Anacardiaceae, Leguminosae)
5. Ego – weak/strong. (Rubiaceae, Cucurbitaceae, Ranunculaceae, Rosaceae)
6. Guilt/anxiety; conscience/duty – social obligation. (Liliaceae, Berberidaceae, Lauraceae, Papaveraceae, Rutaceae)

Fig. 13.2 Desai's suggested schema

Her suggestion is that in moving up the evolutionary ladder from simpler plants to more complex plants (from fungi to coniferae to flowering plants) the human issues to which the plant families correspond also become more complex. She writes, "So as we go from simpler to complex structures the types of conflicts also become complex. Not only the issues of survival and reproduction will be predominant, but also we may find *emotions, ego, duty, performance or guilt like issues dominating the scene.*"[11]

A schema such as this offers a possible approach. I have included it here simply as a suggested basis for further research. However, the interesting thing is how closely her schema corresponds with the developmental model and the periods of the periodic table that we have already discussed. I've put them alongside each other below:

Desai's suggested schema	Developmental stage	Periodic table series
Dependence for survival and procreation	Intrauterine/birth and physical	First/second
Survival and growth despite strong adversities	Physical	Second
Dependent plus instinctual	Physical	Second
Strong instincts	Physical/Emotional	Second/third
Emotions	Emotional	Third
Identity	Mental/conceptual	Third
Ego – weak/strong	Mental/conceptual	Third
Guilt/anxiety, conscience/duty, social obligation	Rule/role mind	Fourth

Fig. 13.3 Desai, stages of development and periodic table

It may also be possible to work towards a schema for the animal kingdom along similar lines. Such a schema would go, following the line of evolution, from invertebrates to vertebrates. It would go from sea creatures to land dwellers to birds. It could also go from creatures such as arthropods, to molluscs, to reptiles, to mammals.

Patient and journey

When we first go to a homœopath we are asked to notice symptoms. It may be that we have ignored the inner world of sensations and feelings for so long that that this inner life can now only appear to us in the form of troublesome symptoms. Through lack of awareness of the internal activity of the vital force, this dynamic activity has been replaced by settled symptom.

As homœopathic treatment progresses we will probably become freer of symptoms. Fear and pain will have less hold on our minds. Homœopathy is doing its job. But now what? If we can now begin to cultivate the art of attending to, of noticing, the images and sensations of the inner life of the vital force the necessity of becoming stuck or ill decreases. The language of feeling and instinct can now be heard without having to be locked into symptoms. Now we are no longer a patient, but a traveller on the path. We can respond to feelings without them becoming symptoms. We can attend to the ups and downs in the body, noting aches and pains and alterations of rhythm as the movement and wisdom of our physical presence. Minor problems can disappear when we open ourselves to their meaning in this way. They don't need to become settled symptoms. We listen to and feel feelings before they take on a compulsive character. In similar fashion we attend to our dreams; often utterly confused by their content, but sometimes being blessed by insight.

What is it we are witnessing here? We are witnessing the movement from the condition of patient to the condition of patience. This patience involves a patient attention to the different manners of expression of the voice of nature. Signals in the body alert you to what is happening in and around you. Feelings guide you in the stream of life. Intuition tells you more about a situation than logic can. However, most of us ceased to listen a long time ago. We shut out these voices, and they have no choice but to return as symptoms. Illness and learning the art of attention to symptoms is often the first step in one's re-education in the ways of the soul. To tread this path is to acknowledge that one is always in need of guidance, because one is always walking in the dark. When one gives up the old routines of learnt logic, one must find a new logic, a new knowing. In this new knowing one is guided by the soul – not just the individual soul, but the soul of the world. Thus to listen to your own true nature can be none other than to listen to the nature of the world. What other voice could it be that speaks through the cells of your body, the waters of your feelings and the wings of your intuition? Let it be.

Notes

Chapter One

1. Arthur Koestler, *The Ghost in the Machine.*

2. Ken Wilber, *A Brief History of Everything*, and Ken Wilber, *Sex, Ecology, Spirituality: The Spirit of Evolution.*

3. For more on morphic fields, see: Rupert Sheldrake, *The Presence of the Past*, and Edward C. Whitmont, *The Alchemy of Healing: Psyche and Soma.*

For vital force, see: Samuel Hahnemann, *Organon of the Medical Art* (edited O'Reilly).

4. On this subject Hahnemann writes:

"When a person falls ill, it is initially only this spirit-like, autonomic life force (life principle), everywhere present in the organism, that is mistuned through the dynamic influence of a morbific agent inimical to life. Only the life principle, mistuned to such abnormality, can impart to the organism the adverse sensations and induce in the organism the irregular functions that we call disease. The life principle is a power-wesen (ed: dynamic essence) invisible in itself, only discernible by its effects on the organism. Therefore, its morbid mistunement only makes itself known by manifestations of disease in feelings and functions (the only aspects of the organism accessible to the senses of the observer and the medical-art practitioner). In other words, the morbid mistunement of the life principle makes itself discernible by disease symptoms; in no other way can it make itself known."

Samuel Hahnemann, *Organon of the Medical Art* (edited O'Reilly), aphorism 11.

5. Reference to the objective psyche is found throughout the work of Jung and Jungians. See for example: C. G. Jung, *Psychology and Alchemy*, and Anthony Stevens, *Private Myths: Dreams and Dreaming*, p. 204.

Chapter Two

1. Edward C. Whitmont, *The Alchemy of Healing: Psyche and Soma*, p. 104.

2. Mircea Eliade suggests that the Sun, as distinct from the Moon, which stands for ebb and flow, stands for an unchanging consciousness. He says that many heroic mythologies are solar in nature. See: Mircea Eliade, *The Sacred and the Profane.*

Eliade is quoted on the subject of solar consciousness and the hero, in: Anne Baring and Jules Cashford, *The Myth of the Goddess: Evolution of an Image*, p. 290.

3. For example, Chiron, the leader of the centaurs and teacher of heroes and gods such as Heracles and Asclepius, sustained an unhealing wound from a poisoned arrow loosed from the bow of Heracles.

4. In his book, Secrets of the Talking Jaguar, Martin Prechtel describes his life as a shaman in a Mayan village in Guatemala. The book contains fine accounts of the relationship of dreams and healing to the world of invisible powers: Martin Prechtel, *Secrets of the Talking Jaguar.*

5. Bede Griffiths, *A New View of Reality: Western Science, Eastern Mysticism and Christian Faith*, p. 70.

6. For more on this see Erich Neumann's monumental work: Erich Neumann, *The Origins and History of Consciousness*.

7. For an outline of these developments as viewed by orthodox anthropology, see: Richard Leakey, *The Origin of Humankind*.

8. Anne Baring and Jules Cashford, *The Myth of the Goddess: Evolution of an Image*.

9. Erich Neumann, *The Origins and History of Consciousness*, pp. XIX, 268.

10. See Joseph Campbell's classic work: Joseph Campbell, *The Hero with a Thousand Faces*.

11. J. T. Kent, *Lectures on Homœopathic Philosophy*, chapter XIX.

12. Samuel Hahnemann, *Organon of the Medical Art* (edited O'Reilly), footnote to aphorism 22.

Chapter Three

1. Barbara G. Walker, *The Woman's Encyclopedia of Myths and Secrets*.

2. This story is told by Plato as the "Myth of Er" in book ten of *The Republic*.

For more on the Fates see: Robert Graves, *The Greek Myths*.

3. For more on the soul's destiny and the Fates, see the work of leading archetypal psychologist, James Hillman: James Hillman, *The Soul's Code: In Search of Character and Calling*.

4. Ken Wilber, *A Brief History of Everything*, and Ken Wilber, *Sex, Ecology, Spirituality: The Spirit of evolution*.

5. Stanislav Grof. *The Holotropic Mind: The Three Levels of Human Consciousness and how they Shape our Lives*.

6. Harry van der Zee. *Miasms in Labour*.

7. A good example of important research in this field is Margaret Mahler's work: Margaret S. Mahler, *The Psychological Birth of the Human Infant: Symbiosis and Individuation*, p. 54.

8. Ken Wilber, *A Brief History of Everything*, p.165.

9. Wilber draws heavily on the work of the Swiss researcher Jean Piaget. Piaget identifies four fundamental developmental stages. They are typical and universal stages in the continuum of development. However, the way and speed in which a child moves through these stages will vary with cultural and environmental conditions. The four stages are:

Sensorimotor; 0 - 2 years
Pre-operational; 2 -7 years
Concrete operational; 7 - 11 years
Formal operational; 11 - 15 years

See: Jean Piaget, *The Essential Piaget* (eds., H. Gruber and J. Voneche), and Richard D. Gross, *Psychology: The Science of Mind and Behaviour*.

10. Concerning the fundamental structures of consciousness, Wilber draws on the work of Jean Gebser: Jean Gebser, *The Ever-Present Origin*.

11. Ken Wilber, *A Brief History of Everything*, p. 169.

12. The concept of the shadow is spoken of throughout the works of Jung and the Jungians. See for example: C. G. Jung, *Man and his Symbols*.

13. These terms come from the work of cognitive-developmental theorist, Lawrence Kohlberg. For an introduction to his work, see: Richard D. Gross, *Psychology: The Science of Mind and Behaviour*.

14. For more on this figure see: Ken Wilber, *A Brief History of Everything*.

Richard D. Gross, *Psychology: The Science of Mind and Behaviour*.

Abraham Maslow, *The Farther Reaches of Human Nature*.

Samuel Hahnemann, *Organon of the Medical Art*, aphorism 5.

Chapter Four

1. Jan Scholten, *Homœopathy and the Elements*.

2. Jeremy Sherr, *The Homœopathic Proving of Hydrogen*.

3. Rajan Sankaran, *The Substance of Homœopathy*, p.141.

4. S. R. Phatak, *Materia Medica of Homœopathic Medicines*.

5. Elizabeth Wright Hubbard, "Mental Portraits of Remedies familiar and Unfamiliar", *Homœopathy*, January - February 1984.

6. Jan Scholten, *Homœopathy and Minerals*, and Jan Scholten, *Homœopathy and the Elements*.

7. Frans Vermeulen, *Prisma: The Arcana of Materia Medica Illuminated*.

8. S.R. Phatak, *Materia Medica of Homœopathic Medicines*.

9. Rajan Sankaran, *The Substance of Homœopathy*, p.134.

10. Rajan Sankaran, *The Soul of Remedies*, p.124.

11. Edward C. Whitmont, *Psyche and Substance: Essays on Homeopathy in the Light of Jungian Psychology*, p.126.

12. Rajan Sankaran, *The Soul of Remedies*.

13. This observation from Vithoulkas is noted in: Frans Vermeulen, *Synoptic Materia Medica*.

14. Kent refers to this in his lecture on Magnesia carbonica: J.T. Kent, *Lectures on Homœopathic Materia Medica*.

15. Jan Scholten, *Homœopathy and the Elements*.

16. Rajan Sankaran, *The Soul of Remedies*, pp. 3,4.

17. Richard Leakey, *The Origin of Humankind*, pp. 36-41.

18. George Vithoulkas, *The Essence of Materia Medica*.

19. T.S. Eliot, *Collected Poems 1909-1962*.

20. All symptoms listed in this chapter are taken from *The Complete Repertory: Millennium Edition* (CD).

21. Wilber sees this as a one, two, three process in which the self steps up to and identifies with a new stage, then begins to move beyond and dis-identify with that stage, and, in the third phase identifies with the next stage of development. See: Ken Wilber, *A Brief History of Everything*, pp. 144,145.

Jean Piaget, whose pioneering work Wilber particularly draws on, suggests that each stage is characterised by accommodation, assimilation, equilibrium and disequilibrium. In other words the self has to accommodate to a new range of experiences. It has to assimilate and adapt. It achieves a posture of stability and balance at the new stage. New demands then lead to disequilibrium, which initiates a new cycle of growth. For an introduction to Piaget's work see: Richard D. Gross, *Psychology: The Science of Mind and Behaviour*.

22. Jan Scholten, *Homœopathy and the Elements*.

23. Sankaran says that the main feeling of Iodum and the other halogens is one of betrayal. See: Rajan Sankaran, *The Substance of Homœopathy*, pp. 149,152.

Chapter Five

1. Frans Vermeulen, *Concordant Materia Medica*.

2. Edward Whitmont has suggested that Phosphorus is concerned with the phenomenon of "inner light" (consciousness, wisdom, intellect), as well as the phenomenon of chemical luminescence. See: Edward C. Whitmont, *Psyche and Substance: Essays on Homeopathy in the Light of Jungian Psychology*.

3. Catherine R. Coulter, *Portraits of Homœopathic Medicines: Psychological Analysis of Selected Constitutional Types*, p.8.

4. *The Bible* (King James version), Isaiah, chapter 14, verses 12-17.

5. This observation from Vithoulkas is noted in: Frans Vermeulen, *Synoptic Materia Medica*.

6. Jan Scholten, *Homœopathy and the Elements*.

7. Frans Vermeulen, *Synoptic Materia Medica*.

8. Rajan Sankaran, *The Soul of Remedies*.

9. Anne Baring and Jules Cashford, *The Myth of the Goddess: Evolution of an Image*, pp. 285-290.

10. Rajan Sankaran, *The Soul of Remedies*.

11. See note 13 for Chapter 3, which refers to the work of Lawrence Kohlberg.

12. Jan Scholten, *Homœopathy and the Elements*.

13. *The Columbia Electronic Encyclopedia*.

14. S.R. Phatak, *Materia Medica of Homœopathic Medicines*.

15. Rajan Sankaran, *The Soul of Remedies*.

16. Frans Vermeulen, *Concordant Materia Medica*.

17. Jan Scholten, *Homœopathy and the Elements*.

18. Jan Scholten, *Homœopathy and the Elements*.

19. Jan Scholten, *Homœopathy and the Elements*.

20. Rajan Sankaran, *The Soul of Remedies*.

21. Wihelm Pelikan, *The Secrets of Metals*, p.99.

22. Rajan Sankaran, *The Soul of Remedies*.

23. Frans Vermeulen, *Concordant Materia Medica*.

24. Jan Scholten, *Homœopathy and the Elements*.

25. Wihelm Pelikan, *The Secrets of Metals*.

26. Rajan Sankaran, *The Soul of Remedies*.

27. Jan Scholten, *Homœopathy and the Elements*.

28. Divya Chabra, Lecture on remedies of the sixth period of the periodic table, Mumbai, February 2002.

29. Jan Scholten, *Homœopathy and the Elements*.

30. Joseph Campbell, *The Hero with a Thousand Faces*.

31. Mircea Eliade, *Shamanism: Archaic Techniques of Ecstasy*.

32. Jeremy Sherr, *The Homœopathic Proving of Plutonium nitricum*.

33. Catherine Sharfstein, "I am in a dark tunnel..." *The Homœopath*, No. 76., Winter 2000, p.48.

34. Jan Scholten, *Homœopathy and the Elements*.

35. Alexander Roob, *Alchemy and Mysticism*, pp. 38, 41.

Chapter Six

1. Jeremy Sherr calls this dynamic activity of the vital force the "verb." "Pressing" is a verb. It describes the individual's consciousness of the activity of the vital force. It describes the activity of the vital force (dynamis) impinging on consciousness and thus drawing attention to itself. It is "pressing", Sherr says, that we should be attentive to. If I ignore the pressing in my chest for long enough I could end up with a pathological respiratory dysfunction, asthma. The "verb" has now taken a pathological form. As a symptom "pressing" is more significant than difficult respiration. It represents the problem as it reveals itself in con-sciousness. See: Jeremy Sherr, *Dynamic Materia Medica: Syphilis, p. 9.*

2. James Hillman, *Healing Fiction*, pp. 97-100.

3. J.T. Kent, *New Remedies, Clinical Cases, Lesser Writings, Aphorisms and Precepts*, pp. 274.

4. J.T. Kent, *New Remedies, Clinical Cases, Lesser Writings, Aphorisms and Precepts*, pp. 275.

5. C.M. Boger, preface to *Boenninghausen's Characteristics and Repertory* (translated, compiled and augmented by C.M. Boger).

6. S.R. Phatak, *Materia Medica of Homœopathic Medicines*.

7. Rajan Sankaran, *The Substance of Homœopathy*.

8. The idea of projection is fundamental to the psychological theory of Jung and those who have followed him. See for example: Jung. C. G., *The Psychology of the Transference*.

9. Samuel Hahnemann, *Organon of the Medical Art* (edited O'Reilly).

10. Reactions are equal and opposite to sensations. A sensation of tightness produces an equal and opposite action to relieve tightness. Thus the modality (relief from loosening) is also equal and opposite to the sensation. See: Rajan Sankaran, *An Insight into Plants*.

11. Kent frequently refers to the "economy." For example he writes, "It is the sole duty of the physician to heal the sick. It is not his sole duty to heal the results of sickness, but the sickness itself. When the man himself has been restored to health, there will be restored harmony in the tissues and in the activities. Then the sole duty of the physician is to put in order the interior of the economy, i.e., the will and understanding conjoined." J.T. Kent, *Lectures on Homœopathic Philosophy*, p.22.

By his use of the word "economy", I understand him to mean the dynamic movement of incomings and outgoings on the levels of mind, emotions and body. In a sense the mind/body organism *is* the activity of what is coming in, being processed and being discharged. In other words the human being is a verb, not a noun. This "dynamic activity" or "economy" needs to be in a healthy balance.

12. Freud wrote frequently about this dynamic with reference to human psychology. See: Sigmund Freud, *Two Short Accounts of Psycho-Analysis*.

Chapter 7

1. Samuel Hahnemann, *The Chronic Diseases*, p.28.

2. Samuel Hahnemann, *Organon of the Medical Art* (edited O'Reilly), entry "itch diathesis" in the glossary.

3. Genital figwarts are, according to Hahnemann, the hallmark of sycosis. The word sycosis comes from the Greek, *sukosis*, meaning fig-like. Sycosis follows the urethral infection that we know as gonorrhoea. True gonorrhoea is identified by the presence of the gonococcus, Neisseria gonorrhoea. In the days before bacteriology Hahnemann was able to identify true gonorrhoea by the presence of figwarts. See: Samuel Hahnemann, *Organon of the Medical Art* (edited O'Reilly), entry "Sycosis" in the glossary.

4. Samuel Hahnemann, *The Chronic Diseases* (translated Louis H. Tafel), p.29.

5. Samuel Hahnemann, *The Chronic Diseases* (translated Louis H. Tafel), pp. 36, 37.

6. Samuel Hahnemann, *The Chronic Diseases* (translated Louis H. Tafel), pp. 33, 31.

7. Kent's view is clear from the following: "Psora is the underlying cause, and is the primitive or primary disorder of the human race. It is a disordered state of the internal economy of the human race. This state expresses itself in the forms of the varying chronic diseases, or chronic manifestations. If the human race had remained in a state of perfect order, psora could not have existed. The susceptibility to psora opens out a question altogether too broad to study among the sciences at a medical college. It is all together too extensive, for it goes to the very primitive wrong of the human race, the very first sickness of the human race, that is the spiritual sickness, from which first state the race progressed into what may be called the true susceptibly to psora, which in turn laid the foundation for other diseases." J.T. Kent, *Lectures on Homœopathic Philosophy*, p.126.

Constantine Hering, the forefather of homœopathy in America, and predecessor of Kent, also saw a close identity between the doctrine of original sin and Hahnemann's notion of psora. C. Hering, footnote to his preface to Hahnemann's *The Chronic Diseases* (translated Hempel).

8. J.T. Kent, Lectures on Homœopathic Philosophy, p.134.

9. This is the classification I was taught by my first homœopathic teacher, John Damonte. It is based on the classifications found in:

Proceso Ortega, *Notes on the Miasms*.

10. Rajan Sankaran, *The Soul of Remedies*, p.221.

11. Rajan Sankaran, *The Soul of Remedies*, p.223.

12. Rajan Sankaran, *The System of Homœopathy*, pp. 472, 473.

13. Rajan Sankaran, Seminar, London, 16th, 17th November 2002.

14. Jan Scholten, *Homœopathy and the Elements*.

Scholten places aluminium in vertical column 3. It is normally placed in column 13. He places silicon in column 10. It is normally placed in column 14.

15. Rajan Sankaran, *The Soul of Remedies*.

16. Sankaran's ideas on the miasms have been developed in *The Soul of Remedies* and *The System of Homœopathy*, as well as in lectures delivered in Mumbai, India between 25th January and 6th February 2002.

17. Rajan Sankaran, "The miasm represents the depth and pace of the disease." Seminar, Mumbai, January 2002.

Chapter Eight

1. Nicholas Goodrick - Clarke, *Paracelsus: Essential Readings*.

2. Steiner and other anthroposophists refer to this basic classification throughout their lectures and writings. See for example: Rudolf Steiner, *Occult Physiology*.

3. For example see: Max Heindel, *The Rosicrucian Cosmo-Conception*.

4. Rajan Sankaran, *The Soul of Remedies*, and Chaim Rosenthal, "Kingdoms Understanding in Homœopathy: A New Approach"

Homœopathic Links, Volume 13, Spring 2000, pp. 42-46.

5. Rajan Sankaran, lectures delivered in Mumbai, India, between 25th January and 6th February 2002.

Chapter Nine

1. More about the four functions can be found in any introduction to Jung's work. See for example: Fordham, Frieda. *An Introduction to Jung's Psychology.*

2. Misha Norland (in collaboration with Adam Martanda), *Mappa Mundi and the Dynamics of Change: A Synthesis of the Four Elements and the Four Temperaments*, and Reves, Joseph. *24 Chapters in Homœopathy.*

3. Misha Norland (in collaboration with Adam Martanda), *Mappa Mundi and the Dynamics of Change: A Synthesis of the Four Elements and the Four Temperaments.*

The map appears inconsistent in some respects – for example the time is anticlockwise. This is because the map attempts to synthesise space, time and associated qualities into a single whole. It has its own logic. As a whole it works. Approach it with imagination. Try it!

4. Frans Vermeulen, *Concordant Materia Medica.*

5. Bryonia is listed under many "milk" symptoms, for example:
Generalities; Food and drinks; milk; agg.
Generalities; Food and drinks; milk; aversion
Generalities; Food and drinks; milk; aversion; mothers
Generalities; Food and drinks; milk; desires
Generalities; Food and drinks; milk; desires; warm
Chest; Milk; non-pregnant women
Chest; Milk; absent
Chest; Milk; affected; emotions, from
Chest; Milk; suppressed
Chest; Inflammation; mammae, mastitis
Chest; Inflammation; mammae, mastitis; pregnancy, during, painful
See: *The Complete Repertory: Millennium Edition* (CD).

6. Frans Vermeulen, *Concordant Materia Medica.*

7. See Edward Whitmont's essay on Natrum muriaticum. Edward C. Whitmont, *Psyche and Substance: Essays on Homœopathy in the Light of Jungian Psychology.*

8. Frans Vermeulen, *Concordant Materia Medica.*

9. S.R. Phatak, *Materia Medica of Homœopathic Medicines.*

10. Frans Vermeulen, *Concordant Materia Medica.*

11. Frans Vermeulen, *Concordant Materia Medica.*

12. Rajan Sankaran, *The Soul of Remedies.*

13. Frans Vermeulen, Prisma: *The Arcana of Materia Medica Illuminated*, p. 222

14. Frans Vermeulen, *Concordant Materia Medica.*

15. J.T. Kent, *Lectures on Homœopathic Materia Medica.*

16. Frans Vermeulen, *Concordant Materia Medica.*

17. Jung called the centre that transcends and includes conflicting opposites the "transcendent function." The stance of this centre is higher and more inclusive than the existing conflicting positions. He wrote of it in *The Structure and Dynamics of the Psyche* (Collected Works: Volume 8). See: Joseph Campbell (editor), *The Portable Jung.*

18. Richard Wilhelm (translation), *I Ching: Book of Changes.*

Chapter Ten

1. Non physical frequencies such as those of sound can produce substantial effects. If sand is placed on a metal sheet and vibrations equivalent to musical tones (produced by a crystal oscillator) are passed through the sheet, different rhythmic patterns will form on the sheet. See: Hans Jenny, *Cymatics: The Structure and Dynamics of Waves and Vibrations.*

2. Richard D. Gross, *Psychology: The Science of Mind and Behaviour*, p.153.

3. Hahnemann sites examples of natural diseases being cured by other natural diseases, having similar symptoms. See: Samuel Hahnemann, *Organon of the Medical Art* (edited O'Reilly), aphorism 46.

4. Rupert Sheldrake, *The Presence of the Past*, pp. 108, 109.

5. C. G. Jung, *The Archetypes and the Collective Unconscious* (Collected Works, volume 9, part 1), paragraph 99.

6. Joseph Campbell, *The Masks of God: Primitive Mythology*, pp. 296, 297.

7. Such rituals expressed the understanding of all first peoples that anything taken from nature must be paid for, that sacrifices must be made in an attempt to keep man's activities in harmony with the whole. In killing an antelope such people understood that the wholeness of nature was being violated, and that only by aligning themselves with the intentions of the whole, by constantly recalling that man is here as the servant of nature and not for his own ends, could the effects of such necessary violations be offset. See: Joseph Campbell, *The Masks of God: Primitive Mythology*, chapter 7.

8. It is from these rituals that theatre and drama evolved, with the witnesses of the sacred drama becoming the audience in modern theatre. See: Barbara G. Walker, *The Woman's Encyclopedia of Myths and Secrets*.

9. Samuel Hahnemann, *Organon of the Medical Art* (edited O'Reilly), aphorism 31.

10. Robert Sardello, *Freeing the Soul from Fear*.

11. J.T. Kent, *Lectures on Homœopathic Philosophy*, p.106.

Chapter Eleven

1. Jeremy Sherr, *The Dynamics and Methodology of Homœopathic Provings*.

2. Nicholas Goodrick - Clarke, *Paracelsus: Essential Readings*, p.129.

3. William Gutman, *Homœopathy: The Fundamentals of its Philosophy, the Essence of its Remedies*.

4. Much on this subject can be found in the anthroposophical literature. See for example: Rudolf Steiner, *Goethean Science*, and Ralph Twentyman, *The Science and Art of Healing*, Chapter 7.

5. Samuel Hahnemann, *Organon of Medicine* (translated by R.E. Dudgeon and William Boericke), preface to the second edition.

6. Samuel Hahnemann, *Organon of Medicine* (translated by R.E. Dudgeon and William Boericke), preface to the second edition.

7. Hahnemann referred to these actions as *initial action* and *after-action* or *counter-action*. See: Samuel Hahnemann, *Organon of the Medical Art* (edited O'Reilly), aphorisms 62 - 66.

8. Misha Norland, "Group and Proving Phenomena", *The Homœopath*, No. 72., Winter 1999, pp. 38 - 41.

9. This is Abraham Maslow's term for breakthrough transpersonal experiences. See: Abraham Maslow, *The Farther Reaches of Human Nature*.

10. Misha Norland, "Group and Proving Phenomena", *The Homœopath*, No. 72., Winter 1999, pp. 38 - 41.

11. Samuel Hahnemann, *Organon of the Medical Art* (edited O'Reilly), aphorisms 105 - 120.

12. For more on this perspective see the work of Martin Prechtel. He was initiated, as a shaman, into the ancient teachings of a Mayan village in Guatemala. The events (in time and eternity) that he relates took place in and around the village, before the village, its inhabitants and its way of life were crushed by right wing and left wing forces in the 1980's. See: Martin Prechtel, *Secrets of the Talking Jaguar*.

13. Samuel Hahnemann, *Organon of the Medical Art* (edited O'Reilly), footnote to aphorism 141.

14. Samuel Hahnemann, *Organon of the Medical Art* (edited O'Reilly), footnote to aphorism 141.

15. Joseph Campbell, *The Masks of God: Primitive Mythology*, p. 251.

16. Mircea Eliade, *Shamanism: Archaic Techniques of Ecstasy*, p. 36.

17. Marie-Louise von Franz, *Alchemy: An Introduction to the Symbolism and the Psychology*.

18. Michael Emmans Dean, "Homœopathy and Alchemy: (1) A Pharmacological Gold Standard", *The Homœopath*, No. 79., Autumn 2000, p.22.

19. C. G. Jung, *Psychology and Alchemy*, paragraphs 345, 346.

20. Misha Norland, "Group and Proving Phenomena", *The Homœopath*, No. 72., Winter 1999, pp. 38 - 41.

21. Misha Norland, *The Homœopathic Proving of Positronium: A Remedy Prepared from the Annihilation Radiation of Positronium* (an atomic structure consisting of an electron and a positron).

22. In an article for the Journal of Analytical Psychology, Edward Whitmont quotes from one of the great alchemical sources, *The Golden Work of Hermes Trismegistus (Tractataus Aureus)*, by the legendary Hermes Trismegistus. The quote runs thus:

"Now the Bodies of the Metals, are the Domiciles of their Spirits; which when they are received by the Bodies, their terrestrial substance is by little and little made thein [sic], extended and Purified and by their Vivifying Power the Life and Fire, hitherto lying Dormant, is excited and stirred up. For the life which dwells in the Metals, is laid as it were asleep, nor can it exert its Power, or shew it self, unless the Bodies be first Dissolved, Exalted, and turned into Spirit, (for that the Spirit does only Vivifie;) being brought to this Degree of purity and spirituality, and at length to perfection, by their abundant Virtue, they communicate their tinging property to the other imperfect Bodies, and Transmute them into a fixed and permanent substance. This is the property of our Medicine, into which the Bodies are reduced; that at first, one part thereof will tinge ten parts of an imperfect body; then an hundred, after a thousand, then ten thousand, and so infinitely on. By which the Efficacy of the Creator's Word is apparently Evident, Crescite et Multiplicamini, encrease and multiply. And by how much the oftner the medicine is dissolved, by so much the more it encreases in Virtue and Power, which otherwise without any more solutions, would remain in its simple or single State of imperfection: Here is a Celestial and Divine Fountain set Open, which no man is able to draw dry, nor can it be wholly exhausted, should the World endure to External Generations." See: Edward C. Whitmont, "Homœopathy and the Treatment of Borderline Cases", *Journal of Analytical Psychology*, No. 41, 1996, pp. 369 - 386.

The Golden Work of Hermes Trismegistus (1692) was translated from Hebrew to Arabic, then into Greek, then into Latin. An English version was claused and commented upon by William Salmon, professor of Physick, and printed for J. Harris and T. Hawkins. Dr. Whitmont had a private copy of chapter 7, p. 51.

23. Daniel Goleman, *Emotional Intelligence: Why it can matter more than IQ*, chapter 11.

Chapter 12

1. Samuel Hahnemann, *Organon of the Medical Art* (edited O'Reilly), aphorism 8.

2. This snake is often depicted in homœopathic literature as a terrifying aggressive brute. In fact, although amongst the largest of venomous snakes, it is apparently shy and slow to take offence. Its reputation is more to do with human projection than fact. See: Frans Vermeulen, *Prisma: The Arcana of Materia Medica Illuminated.*

3. Constantine Hering records his observations concerning the direction of cure in his preface to Hahnemann's *The Chronic Diseases.* These observations have since become known as Hering's Law of Cure. See: Samuel Hahnemann, *The Chronic Diseases* (translated and edited by Charles J. Hempel), preface. This preface is reprinted in: *The Homœopath*, vol. 7, no. 1, pp. 4 - 11.

4. Samuel Hahnemann, *The Chronic Diseases* (translated Louis H. Tafel), pp. 78 - 79.

5. Samuel Hahnemann, *Organon of the Medical Art* (edited O'Reilly), entry "itch diathesis" in the glossary.

6. Samuel Hahnemann, *The Chronic Diseases* (translated Louis H. Tafel), p. 36, footnote.

7. Samuel Hahnemann, *The Chronic Diseases* (translated Louis H. Tafel). Reference to the effects of this suppression is made throughout the text.

8. This is suggested throughout the text of *The Chronic Diseases.* See for example: Samuel Hahnemann, *The Chronic Diseases* (translated Louis H. Tafel), pp. 44 - 47.

9. J.T. Kent, *Lectures on Homœopathic Philosophy*, pp. 134 - 136.

10. Deepak Chopra describes the elaborate sensitivity and responsiveness of the skin. See CD: Deepak Chopra, *Magical Mind Magical Body: Mastering the Mind/Body Connection for Perfect Health and Total Well-being*.

11. Paul D. Maclean. *A Triune Concept of the Brain and Behaviour*.

12. Anthony Stevens, *Private Myths: Dreams and Dreaming*, p. 102.

13. George Vithoulkas discusses the structural and functional relationships between different organs and systems in the organism. He suggests that such affinities might be based on the common origin of organs and systems (such as skin and nervous system) in one or other of the primary tissue layers – ectoderm, endoderm and mesoderm. See: George Vithoulkas, *The Science of Homœopathy*, chapter 3.

14. *Black's Medical Dictionary*.

15. Margaret S. Mahler, *The Psychological Birth of the Human Infant: Symbiosis and Individuation*, p. 52. For a more general discussion of this developmental stage, see also: Ken Wilber, *A Brief History of Everything*, chapter 10.

16. Robert Sardello, *Love and the Soul: Creating a Future for the Earth*, pp. 94 - 95.

17. Samuel Hahnemann, *The Chronic Diseases* (translated Louis H. Tafel), p.35.

Chapter 13

1. This term became famous through the teachings of George Vithoulkas. The essence of a remedy is a kind of distillation of its essential characteristics. It is the hub of the wheel of which the symptoms are the spokes. See: George Vithoulkas, *The Essence of Materia Medica*.

2. This is Sankaran's term for the fundamental illusion that permeates someone's experience of self or life. For example if a person feels bullied, without rights, then the central delusion could be "persecuted." See: Rajan Sankaran, *The Spirit of Homœopathy*.

3. Samuel Hahnemann, *Organon of the Medical Art* (edited O'Reilly), aphorism 141 and footnote to aphorism 141.

4. Samuel Hahnemann, *Organon of the Medical Art* (edited O'Reilly), footnote to aphorism 84.

5. According to Arnold Mindell (founder of Process Orientated Psychology) the dreambody is the entity expressing itself through both dreams and physical phenomena. His notion of the dreambody is very similar to Hahnemann's concept of the vital force. For Mindell the dreambody manifests through various channels or modes of perception and/or activity. During deep therapeutic work the dreambody can switch channels, moving, for example, from image, to feeling, to sensation, to motion and back again. See: Arnold Mindell, *Working with the Dreaming Body*.

6. Rajan Sankaran has proposed a four level model of case taking. It maps four levels, from the surface level – recording, observation – to the deepest level in which delusions, feelings, sensations, actions and modalities coalesce into a unified picture. See: Rajan Sankaran, *The System of Homœopathy*.

7. Rajan Sankaran, lectures delivered in Mumbai, India, between 25th January and 6th February 2002.

8. Rajan Sankaran, *The Soul of Remedies*. Rajan Sankaran, *An Insight into Plants* (Vols. 1 and 2).

9. Rajan Sankaran, *An Insight into Plants* (Vols. 1 and 2).

10. S.R. Phatak, *Materia Medica of Homœopathic Medicines*.

11. Rupal Desai, *Our Magnificent Plants*, p. 320.

Bibliography

Homœopathy

Boenninghausen, Carl von. Boenninghausen's Characteristics and Repertory (translated, compiled and augmented by C.M. Boger), M.V. Kulkarni for Roy and Co., Bombay, 1936.

Coulter, Catherine R., *Portraits of Homœopathic Medicines: Psychological Analyses of Selected Homœopathic Constitutional Types*, North Atlantic Books, Berkley, California, 1986.

Dean, Michael Emmans. "Homœopathy and Alchemy: (1) A Pharmacological Gold Standard", *The Homœopath* (Journal of the Society of Homœopaths), No. 79, Northampton, 2000.

Desai, Rupal. Our Magnificent Plants, Rupal Desai, Mumbai, 2002.

Gutman, William. *Homœopathy: The Fundamentals of its Philosophy, The Essence of its Remedies*, Homœopathic Medical Publishers, Bombay, 1978.

Hahnemann, Samuel. *The Chronic Diseases: Their Peculiar Nature and Their Homœopathic Cure* (Theoretical part; translated from the second enlarged German edition of 1835, by Louis H. Tafel), Jain Publishing Co., New Delhi.

Hahnemann, Samuel. *The Chronic Diseases: Their Specific Nature and Homœopathic Treatment* (translated and edited by Charles J. Hempel). William Radde, New York, 1845.

Hahnemann, Samuel. *Organon of the Medical Art*, (Edited and annotated by Wenda Brewster O'Reilly and translated by Steven Decker: adapted from the sixth edition of the *Organon der Heilkunst* completed by Samuel Hahnemann in 1842), Birdcage Books, Redmond, Washington, 1996.

Hahnemann, Samuel. *Organon of Medicine* (translated from the fifth edition by R.E. Dudgeon, with additions and alterations as per the sixth edition translated by William Boericke), Roy Publishing House, Calcutta, 1961.

Hering, Constantine. "Preface to Hahnemann's The Chronic Diseases" (translated Hempel), *The Homœopath* (Journal of the Society of Homœopaths), vol. 7, no. 1, Northampton, 1987.

Kent, James Tyler. *Lectures on Homœopathic Materia Medica: with New Remedies*, Jain Publishing Company, New Delhi, 1972, 1974, 1975.

Kent, James Tyler. *Lectures on Homœopathic Philosophy*, Thorsons, Wellingborough, Northamptonshire, 1979 (original publication of these lectures was 1900).

Kent, James Tyler. *New Remedies, Clinical Cases, Lesser Writings, Aphorisms and Precepts*, B. Jain Publishers, New Delhi, 1980.

Norland, Misha. "Group and Proving Phenomena", *The Homœopath* (Journal of the Society of Homœopaths), No. 72, Northampton, 1999.

Norland, Misha (in collaboration with Adam Martanda). *Mappa Mundi and the Dynamics of Change: A Synthesis of the Four Elements and the Four Temperaments*, School Of Homœopathy (Yondercott House, Uffculme, Devon EX15, 3DR), 2001.

Norland, Misha. "Notes on the Theory of Miasms" (essay), The School of Homœopathy, Devon.

Norland, Misha. "The Homœopathic Proving of Positronium: A Remedy Prepared from the Annihilation Radiation of Positronium (an atomic structure consisting of an electron and a positron)", The School of Homœopathy, Devon, 1998. (The proving report is available on the school's website: www. homeopathyschool.com)

Ortega, Proceso Sanchez. *Notes on the Miasms*, National Homœopathic Pharmacy, New Delhi, 1980.

Phatak, S. R. *Materia Medica of Homœopathic Medicines*, Indian Books and Periodicals Syndicate, New Delhi, 1977.

Reves, Joseph. *24 Chapters in Homœopathy*, Homœopress Ltd., Haifa, Israel, 1993.

Rosenthal, Chaim. "Kingdoms Understanding in Homœopathy: A New Approach", *Homœopathic Links*, The Netherlands, 2000.

Sankaran, Rajan. *The Soul of Remedies*, Homœopathic Medical Publishers, Mumbai, 1997.

Sankaran, Rajan. *An Insight into Plants (Vols. 1 and 2)*, Homœopathic Medical Publishers, Mumbai, 2002.

Sankaran, Rajan. *The Spirit of Homœopathy*, Dr. Rajan Sankaran, Bombay, 1991.

Sankaran, Rajan. *The Substance of Homœopathy*, Homœopathic Medical Publishers, Bombay, 1994.

Sankaran, Rajan. *The System of Homœopathy*, Homœopathic Medical Publishers, Mumbai, 2000.

Sharfstein, Catherine. "I am in a dark tunnel...", *The Homœopath* (Journal of the Society of Homœopaths), No. 76, Northampton, 2000.

Sherr, Jeremy. *The Dynamics and Methodology of Homœopathic Provings*, Dynamis Books, West Malvern, 1994.

Sherr, Jeremy. *Dynamic Materia Medica: Syphilis*, Dynamis Books, Great Malvern, 2002.

Sherr, Jeremy. *The Homœopathic Proving of Hydrogen*, Dynamis School of Homœopathy, Malvern, Worcestershire, 1992.

Sherr, Jeremy. *The Homœopathic Proving of Plutonium nitricum*, Dynamis Books, Malvern, Worcestershire, 1999.

Scholten, Jan. *Homœopathy and the Elements*, Stichting Alonnisoss, Utrecht, 1996.

Scholten, Jan. *Homœopathy and Minerals*, Stichting Alonnisoss, Utrecht, 1993.

Twentyman, Ralph. *The Science and Art of Healing*, Floris Books, Edinburgh, 1989.

Vermeulen, Frans. *Concordant Materia Medica*, Merlijn Publishers, Haarlem, The Netherlands, 1994.

Vermeulen, Frans. *Prisma: The Arcana of Materia Medica Illuminated*, Emryss bv Publishers, Haarlem, The Netherlands, 2002.

Vermeulen, Frans. *Synoptic Materia Medica*, Merlijn Publishers, Haarlem, The Netherlands, 1992.

Vithoulkas, George. *The Essence of Materia Medica*, B. Jain Publishers Ltd., New Delhi, 1988.

Vithoulkas, George. *The Science of Homœopathy*, Grove Press, New York, 1980.

Whitmont, Edward C. "Alchemy, Homœopathy and the Treatment of Borderline Cases", *Journal of Analytical Psychology*, 1996.

Whitmont, Edward C. *Psyche and Substance: Essays on Homœopathy in the Light of Jungian Psychology*, North Atlantic Books, Richmond, California, 1980.

Zandvoort, Roger van. *The Complete Repertory: Millennium Edition* (CD for Macintosh), Institute for Research in Homeopathic Information and Symptomatology, Leidschendam, The Netherlands, 2000.

Zee, Harry van der. *Miasms in Labour*, Alonnissos, Utrecht, 2000.

General

Baring, Anne and Cashford, Jules. *The Myth of the Goddess: Evolution of an Image*, Arkana (Penguin Books), London, 1993.

Black's Medical Dictionary (37th edition edited by Gordon Macpherson), A. and C. Black, London, 1992.

Campbell, Joseph. *The Hero with a Thousand Faces*, Bollingen Series XVII, Princeton University Press, 1972.

Campbell, Joseph. *The Masks of God: Primitive Mythology*, Penguin Books, London, 1976.

Campbell, Joseph (editor). *The Portable Jung*, Penguin Books, Middlesex, 1976.

Chopra, Deepak. *Magical Mind Magical Body: Mastering the Body/Mind Connection for Perfect Health and Total Well-being* (produced on CD), Nightingale Conant, Paignton, Devon, 1990.

Columbia Electronic Encyclopedia (Sixth Edition). Columbia University Press, 2000.

Eliade, Mircea. *Shamanism: Archaic Techniques of Ecstasy*, Arkana (Penguin Books), London, 1989.

Eliade, Mircea. *The Sacred and the Profane* (translated by Willard R. Trask), Harcourt, Brace Jovanovich, New York and London, 1959.

Eliot, T.S. *Collected Poems: 1909 - 1962*, Faber and Faber, London, 1974.

Fordham, Frieda. *An Introduction to Jung's Psychology*, Penguin, Middlesex, 1953.

Freud, Sigmund. *Two Short Accounts of Psycho-Analysis*, Penguin Books, London, 1991.

Gebser, Jean. *The Ever-Present Origin* (translated by Noel Barstad and Algis Mickunas), Ohio University Press, Ohio, 1985.

Goleman, Daniel. *Emotional Intelligence: why it can matter more than IQ*, Bloomsbury, London, 1996.

Goodrick-Clarke, Nicholas. *Paracelsus: Essential Readings* (selected and translated by Nicholas Goodrick-Clarke), Crucible (imprint of Aquarian Press, part of Thorsons Group), Wellingborough, Northamptonshire, 1990.

Graves, Robert. *The Greek Myths*, Penguin Books, London, 1955.

Griffiths, Bede. *A New Vision of Reality: Western Science, Eastern Mysticism and Christian Faith*, Collins, London, 1989.

Grof, Stanislav (with Hal Zina Bennet). *The Holotropic Mind: The Three Levels of Human Consciousness and how they Shape our Lives*, Harper, San Francisco, 1993.

Gross, Richard D. *Psychology: The Science of Mind and Behaviour*, Hodder & Stoughton, London, 1987.

Heindel, Max. *The Rosicrucian Cosmo-Conception: Man's Past Evolution, Present Constitution and Future Development*, L.N. Fowler and Co., Ltd., London, 1973.

Hillman, James. *Healing Fiction*, Station Hill, Barry Town, New York, 1983.

Hillman, James. *The Soul's Code: In Search of Character and Calling*, Random House, New York, 1996.

Jenny, Hans. *Cymatics: The Structure and Dynamics of Waves and Vibrations*, Basilius Press, Basel, 1967.

Jung, G.G. *Man and his Symbols* (conceived and edited by Jung), Picador, London, 1978.

Jung, C.G. *Psychology and Alchemy* (Collected Works, volume 12), Routledge and Kegan Paul, London, 1980.

Jung, C.G. *The Archetypes and the Collective Unconscious* (Collected Works, volume 9, part 1), Routledge and Kegan Paul, London, 1959.

Jung, C.G. *The Psychology of the Transference*, Ark (Routledge), London, 1983.

Koestler, Arthur. *The Ghost in the Machine*, Random House, New York, 1976.

Leakey, Richard. *The Origin of Humankind*, Phoenix (Orion Books), London, 1995.

MacLean, Paul. D. *A Triune Concept of the Brain and Behaviour* (edited T.J. Boag and D. Campbell), University of Toronto Press, 1973.

Mahler, Margaret S; Pine, Fred; Bergmann, Anni. *The Psychological Birth of the Human Infant: Symbiosis and Individuation*, Hutchinson, London, 1975.

Maslow, Abraham. *The Farther Reaches of Human Nature*, Viking Press, New York, 1972.

Mindell, Arnold. *Working with the Dreaming Body*, Arkana (Penguin), London, 1989.

Neumann, Erich. *The Origins and History of Consciousness*, Bollingen Series XLII, Princeton University Press, 1970.

Pelikan, Wilhelm. *The Secrets of Metals* (translated by Charlotte Lebensart), Anthroposophic Press, Spring Valley, New York, 1973.

Piaget, Jean. *The Essential Piaget* (eds., H. Gruber and J. Voneche), Basic Books, New York, 1977.

Prechtel, Martin. *Secrets of the Talking Jaguar*, Element, Shaftesbury, Dorset, 1998.

Roob, Alexander. *Alchemy and Mysticism*, Taschen, Koln, 1997.

Sardello, Robert. *Freeing the Soul from Fear*, Riverhead Books (Penguin Putnam, Inc.), New York, 1999.

Sardello, Robert. *Love and the Soul: Creating a Future for the Earth*, Harperperennial (HarperCollins), New York, 1996.

Sheldrake, Rupert. *The Presence of the Past*, Fontana, London, 1989.

Steiner, Rudolf. *Goethean Science*, Mercury Press, 1989.

Steiner, Rudolf. *Occult Physiology*, Rudolf Steiner Press, 1983.

Stevens, Anthony. *Private Myths: Dreams and Dreaming*, Penguin, London, 1996.

Trismegistus, Hermes. *Tractatus aureus*, Leipzig, 1610.

Walker, Barbara G. *The Woman's Encyclopedia of Myths and Secrets*, HarperSanFrancisco (HarperCollins), San Francisco, 1983.

Whitmont, Edward C. *The Alchemy of Healing: Psyche and Soma*, North Atlantic Books, Berkeley, California, 1993.

Wilber, Ken. *A Brief History of Everything*, *Newleaf* (Gill and Macmillan), Dublin, 1996.

Wilber, Ken. *Sex, Ecology, Spirituality: The Spirit of Evolution*, Shambhala, Boston and London, 1995.

Wilhelm, Richard (translation). *I Ching: Book of Changes*, Routledge and Kegan Paul Ltd., London, 1968.

Index

Notes

Notes

Notes

Notes

Notes

Notes

Notes

Notes

Notes

Notes